DOROTHY A MICHAEL

EMERGENCY PREPAREDNESS

Disaster Planning for Health Facilities

Jerome S. Seliger, PhD
Associate Professor
Health Administration and Public Health
California State University
Northridge, California

Joan Kelley Simoneau, RN, CCRN, CEN, MICN
Director, Ambulatory/Emergency Services
Robert F. Kennedy Medical Center
Hawthorne, California
and
Director, EmergiTrends Consulting Service
Los Angeles, California

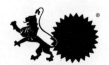

AN ASPEN PUBLICATION®
Aspen Publishers, Inc.

1986

Rockville, Maryland
Royal Tunbridge Wells

Library of Congress Cataloging in Publication Data

Seliger, Jerome S.
Emergency preparedness.

"An Aspen publication."
Includes bibliographies and index.
1. Emergency medical services. 2. Hospitals—Emergency service.
3. Disaster relief—Planning.
I. Simoneau, Joan Kelley. II. Title. III Title: Disaster planning for health
facilities. [DNLM: 1. Disaster Planning—Methods. 2. Health Facilities.
WX 185 S465e]
RA645.5.S45   1986   362.1'8   85-31552
ISBN: 0-87189-290-1

Editorial Services: Ruth Bloom

Library of Congress Catalog Card Number: 85-31552
ISBN: 0-87189-290-1

Printed in the United States of America

1 2 3 4 5

This work is dedicated to the memory of irreplaceable souls who so long ago and far away helped me become: my parents, Julius and Gertrude, brother Harvey, and Aunt Flori; and two who were mentors, Dick Thomas and Katherine Lackey, of Southern Illinois University. They all continue to touch my life.

Jerome S. Seliger

Any endeavor of this magnitude requires a great deal of personal commitment in which family members share. While too young to have been a reviewer, I owe a debt of gratitude to my daughter, Courtney Alyssa, for stray crayon and pen marks on manuscript material, and lost references. She is my great joy, and provided many memories of comic relief under terrific time demands. I also thank my colleagues in emergency nursing for their input and creative thinking over the many years I have been involved in disaster planning for emergency services. I am indebted to the members of my church family for their continued love, support, and genuine acceptance, all of which enable me to produce in my professional life.

Joan Kelley Simoneau

Table of Contents

Acknowledgments   vii

Introduction   ix

Chapter 1—Planning Concepts   1
    What Planning Is   2
    Planning Strategies   4
    Planning Models   5
    Why Plan?   9
    Planning in the Facility: Where It Fits   10
    Who Are the Planners?   13
    Summary   14

Chapter 2—The Planning Process   17
    Step 1: Problem Sensing   17
    Step 2: Goal Setting   20
    Step 3: Needs Assessment   22
    Step 4: Objective Setting   32
    Step 5: Action Plan Detailing   34
    Step 6: Action Implementation   44
    Step 7: Plan Evaluation   44
    Summary   44

Chapter 3—Beginning Work   47
    Patient-Generating Criteria   47
    The Disaster Planning Committee Role   49
    Committee Activities   52
    Hospital and SNF Goals   53

       Linking Community Resources in Planning   57
       Summary   59

Chapter 4—The Disaster Manual **61**
       Model Disaster Manual   63
       Summary   120
       Appendix 4–A   123
       Appendix 4–B   125
       Appendix 4–C   129
       Appendix 4–D   139
       Appendix 4–E   141
       Appendix 4–F   147

Chapter 5—Disaster Preparedness Training and Drills **157**
       Training Modalities   157
       Training Concepts   159
       Barriers to Training   160
       Disaster Training   164
       Attendance at Training Events   171
       Types of Training Programs   172
       Changing the Plan   205
       Learning from the Training Experience   206
       Rewards for Behavior   208
       Summary   212
       Appendix 5–A   215
       Appendix 5–B   222
       Appendix 5–C   224

Chapter 6—Epilogue **229**
       Disaster Stress Syndrome   229
       Victim Response   230
       Handling the Needs of Health Personnel   231
       Emerging Trends in Disaster Experiences   234

Index **241**

Acknowledgments

The authors wish to acknowledge the significant assistance provided by Ms. Virginia Lewis in preparing numerous drafts of this text. Her insightful suggestions regarding form and concept were invaluable and her calm demeanor of immeasurable support in balancing our often high-powered discussions regarding content and flow. We wish also to thank Roy and Pat Azarnoff for use of their office space on many occasions. We finally wish to acknowledge our respective institution for their support of this academic and professional accomplishment.

Introduction

Friday, 5 A.M., . . . a huge oil tanker explodes while offloading cargo in the Los Angeles Harbor, killing four and injuring 50.

Early morning November 21, a fire breaks out in the largest hotel-casino in Las Vegas . . . it spreads quickly throughout the entire ground floor. Two hundred persons are trapped in high-rise towers. Helicopters pluck dozens from balconies and the roof . . . 84 die and more than 700 are injured.

A pleasant spring afternoon in Kansas City, 1,000 people are enjoying a tea dance when a walkway collapses on the dancers below, killing more than 100 and injuring 200.

Dark is settling on a snowy Washington, D.C., when a jet carrying passengers to Florida loses power immediately after leaving the runway and crashes into the 14th Street bridge before plunging into the icy river. Cars, bumper to bumper during the evening rush hour, are crushed. Five persons on the plane survive . . . all others aboard, and several on the bridge, perish.

It's Saturday and families and children enjoy hamburgers at a fast-food restaurant . . . 90 minutes later, 21 are dead, slain by a lone gunman who enters the restaurant and begins shooting without warning or apparent motive. Dozens are injured and in shock, leaving the small town "the saddest town in the nation" (*Los Angeles Times*).

The spring thaw is earlier and more severe than usual. . . . Floods throughout the Ohio River Valley force thousands from their homes . . . inundate hospitals and nursing homes . . . sap Red Cross resources. . . . Elderly patients are evacuated in freezing rain at dawn. . . .

America experiences hundreds of natural and man-made disasters every year. They kill and injure scores of persons and cause tens of thousands to seek emergency care and shelter. But when "ordinary" accidents such as multivehicle crashes, apartment building fires, and industrial accidents also are considered, the probability is high that every health facility can expect some sort of disaster-related experience in any year, regardless of locale.

A disaster situation is an uncontrollable, unexpected, psychologically shocking event. People become victims in an instant and, by acts beyond their individual control, have their fate intimately connected to the fate of others. Every disaster is unique and affects health facilities in unique ways. The time of day, the cause, the scope, the impact, and the duration of the event; prior readiness of facility personnel, equipment, and procedures; and the extent to which institutions collaborate with one another all are variables affecting response to a disaster.

Regardless of disaster type, health facilities are expected to receive victims and survivors and to provide assistance to rescuers. This certainly is the case for hospitals, but also is true for skilled nursing facilities. An external disaster such as a flood or industrial accident requires responses that are no less trying than the urgencies of a fire in the institution itself. Facilities must mobilize quickly and efficiently to meet any sudden demands placed on them.

Disaster planning is *the* means for anticipating disaster. Its purpose is not to reduce the likelihood of disaster; by definition, disaster is an uncontrollable event. Rather, disaster planning seeks to enable rescuers to respond effectively and efficiently regardless of disruption. A disaster imposes unexpected demands for which most people, health care professionals and lay people alike, are inexperienced. Effective plans are plans that work. In the case of disaster planning, the ultimate test is the way in which health care personnel respond to crises attendant to disaster.

The scientific term for effective response to crisis is "adaptive behavior." Behavior that is disorganized and chaotic during a disaster is "maladaptive" and often contributes to increased mortality and morbidity.

A crisis situation disrupts normal life. The impact can be as great for organizations as it is for individuals. In the case of a hospital, a disaster can affect patient care routines, patient mix and census, the use of part or all of the facility, and the quality of care. For individuals, disaster can mean trauma, loss or fear of loss, and for some, onset of anomie—the feeling that norms and social convention are so disrupted that normal life never will be possible again.

Disaster planning goes a long way toward helping facilities and individuals (both health care personnel and consumers) manage the outcomes of disaster. There is a clear relationship between the extent of planning and preparedness training and effective response.

A disaster event that affects many people has quite an impact—different from that which an individual may feel from the death of a spouse, for example. Individuals develop coping mechanisms to handle loss and grief. Communities rarely have such mechanisms. When a sudden large-scale disaster occurs, the community depends on institutional response. Concerned and prepared hospitals and skilled nursing facilities (SNFs) are a crucial component of that response. If they respond ineffectively, the disaster's disruptive effects will be many times greater.

Planning is the process by which people learn to conceptualize their world, understand events in their lives, set goals, and achieve them. This process entails rational thought undertaken with free will, incorporating the ability to imagine future events and invoke appropriate behavior to control them. Yet the disaster planner has no control over the occurrence, magnitude, and extent of a disaster, so disaster planning must focus on survival responses to situations initially beyond human control, and on the moment-to-moment decision making crucial to reorganization of family, community, and society as a whole.

Because they are considered the locus of community care, hospitals and related health care facilities are the first places citizens think of turning to in a disaster. They go there for medical aid, information, emotional support, food and water, and in general because the health facility represents stability and solidity in an otherwise disorganized and unreal world . . . the world of the disaster event.

Emergency Preparedness: Disaster Planning for Health Facilities provides a practical approach to developing and testing a disaster plan. In the first of six chapters, the planning concept is examined from different perspectives including strategies and models and who should be responsible for disaster planning in hospitals and skilled nursing facilities. Included in Chapter 2 are a description of planning as a seven-step process and the details of methods for developing the steps. Chapter 3 specifies roles and activities for a Disaster Planning Committee, goal setting methods for disaster plan development and linkages with community resources. The fourth chapter details thirteen components of a Disaster Manual— examples of each component and recommendations for preparing them. Disaster training methods and programs including drills, simulations, and methods for evaluating the training event are described in Chapter 5. In an Epilogue, disaster stress, the psychological needs of health personnel during an emergency, and trends in emergency preparedness are discussed. The book also makes extensive use of tables, charts, and checklists.

The intent of *Emergency Preparedness* is to provide health organizations with a guide for planning and for training personnel to respond appropriately. Disaster plans are readiness documents. They prescribe action for the duration of a disaster and its immediate aftermath. Effective disaster planning minimizes disruption of services and the emotional trauma that accompanies such an event and assures the best possible medical care, given the situation.

Effective planning can make the difference between early recovery and continuing chaos. It is the authors' hope that this text can serve as a blueprint for action to those entrusted with the responsibility for providing leadership in disaster plan development, plan revision, and preparedness training.

Chapter 1

Planning Concepts

The one value Western man holds in high regard is rationality: subscribing to reason and to the assumption that human beings have the right to improve the world. Most Americans value rationality and expect predictability, confident that the social order—the legal, banking, educational, and health care systems—can be managed to assure quality of life. Rationality involves deductive reasoning, the process of thinking about events broadly at first, then narrowing the focus, comparing events with prior experience, and finally categorizing the events. Most Americans are raised within this conceptual framework.

They are taught to think analytically about the world. Parents, schools, and social institutions reinforce this. By the time children complete kindergarten they know that the adult world values logic more than intuition. They are taught that analysis and deliberation are preferred to feelings and impulse. But valuing "left brain" at the expense of "right brain" judgment may do more harm than good. The two are not inseparable. While logic and deliberation are central to planning, planners should not ignore intuition and feeling; afterall, the human experience invariably is subjective.[1,2]

Human life involves sensing the environment, choosing from among many alternatives, selecting one alternative over another, taking action, and then learning from the experience. Even for the youngest child, living is a reasoning process, i.e., the planning process. Individuals plan what to wear to work, when and what to eat for dinner, where to go on the weekend, etc. Planning is both unconscious and conscious. Everyone plans, including those who proclaim that they hate to plan and never do.

When individuals plan, they usually do so in private and sometimes unconsciously. But planners in organizations such as hospitals and SNFs do their work openly and must involve others. The plans they develop must be put into writing to ensure they are followed routinely and are available for reflection and revision.

Planning makes the assumption that it is possible to control events in the world and that, using reason, people can overcome the most stubborn of problems.

Americans are biased by a cultural message that says they should control events rather than allow events to control them. Mastery of the environment, an expectation basic to planning, is suggested by the Judeo-Christian world view derived from the injunction in Genesis to be fruitful, multiply, and "control. . . ."[3]

This culture carries the normative message that people ought to behave rationally and be responsible for the world in which they live. Thus the planning value is sustained not only by the way people have been taught to think but also by a fundamental societal norm that prescribes control of events as morally right. Given these two factors it would be expected that planning would enjoy ready acceptance, particularly by health professionals who after all are trained in the rationality of the scientific method.

Disaster planning is different from other applications of planning, although the difference is subtle. Disaster planning implies that anyone can be the victim of events beyond personal control and that in the final analysis individuals cannot control the unexpected and uncontrollable, while planning in other cases implies a controllable outcome. It is hardly surprising that people are uncomfortable planning for an uncontrollable event in which they and their loved ones may be victims.

The unique aspect of disaster planning is that it demands that planners reconcile the lack of control in a disaster with the need to plan. While on the one hand the assumption is that planning can make a difference, on the other everyone knows that accidents or "acts of God" are by definition uncontrollable. The result is a subversion of the planning ethic as it applies to disaster planning. Disaster planning is seen by many as superfluous: If disasters are not preventable, why plan? These individuals have difficulty preparing for an inconceivable event. This is as true for health professionals as it is for others.

Disaster planning cannot prevent disasters, but it can limit their consequences. Disaster plans enable survivors to focus rapidly upon and to participate in coordinated response. This aim holds considerable appeal for health care personnel. After all, the mission of their facilities is the provision of care. Sustaining that mission after a disaster can make the process of planning worthwhile, even to those who are skeptical about its necessity.

WHAT PLANNING IS

Planning is a method of evaluating a problem logically, then figuring the best ways to solve it. Planning is synonymous with problem solving. It can be dynamic, a process used to link together those affected by the problem. It also is a way to maximize and coordinate the use of resources. Planning assumptions include:

- There are many possible futures (i.e., there are many solutions to any problem).
- People can use logic to choose the "best" future.
- There are many routes or means for getting to the future of choice.
- It is possible to pick the "best" routes or means.
- It is possible to identify and control impediments that can keep the route or means selected from working.
- People know when they reach the future they want.
- It is possible to anticipate the positive and negative outcomes of a plan.

Each of these, in a very real sense, is a leap of faith. It takes faith in reason and rationality to envision a future and then plan for its achievement.

Plans are only as good as the data they contain, the intent of those who prepare them, and the clarity with which they are written. They are paper or computer versions of what people think they want, nothing more.

As a properly structured intellectual exercise, the planning process can strengthen management decision making and improve collaboration throughout an organization. Planning is the act of preparing a plan, a process that involves examining the present, imagining the future, and prescribing activities for attaining that future. Classical planning occurs in the laboratory all the time. The experimental psychologist, the physiologist, and the biologist, for example, all use the planning process to test hypotheses. In the lab, however, the process of problem solving has many more controllable variables than does the process of problem solving in a situation outside a controlled laboratory setting (Figure 1–1).

For instance, scientists who test an intervention (the independent variable) in a lab have the ability to identify and control intervening variables that may obstruct movement from one point in time to the future (lighting, type of food given subjects, heat, etc.). They also can be very precise in stating in advance what type of future or outcome (the dependent variable) is expected from the planned

Figure 1–1 The Scientific Method as Planning Process

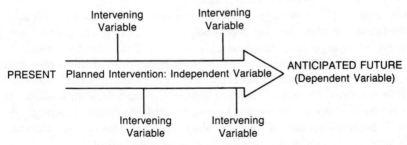

intervention. Hence, the scientists know with some certainty whether the independent variable is responsible for the anticipated outcome. Given time and resources in sufficient amounts, the scientists not only can examine the anticipated outcomes but also can wait for months or years to document discernible unanticipated outcomes.

Even in the laboratory or in controlled clinical studies, however, there are considerable problems and risks. Not infrequently, for instance, drugs and therapeutic regimens once thought to be safe subsequently are determined to have unanticipated side effects, as occurred in the use of DES in the 1950s, Thalidomide a decade later, and the Dalkon Shield and Bendectin in more recent years. Thus, in spite of controlled problem solving, things can and do go wrong.

Outside the laboratory the world is infinitely more complex, with intervening variables more difficult to identify and control and outcomes very difficult to distinguish. While the planning process in that setting mimics the deductive process of the scientific method, there are key differences that health facility planners encounter frequently:

1. It is difficult to achieve consensus regarding the planning goal (the desired future).
2. The "best" intervention approach or route may be difficult to determine because of numerous alternative choices.
3. There are a myriad of intervening variables and it is difficult to determine those that are key, much less control them.
4. It often is difficult to measure the degree to which the plan, once implemented, actually has reached the intended goal.

PLANNING STRATEGIES

A planning strategy is a choice the planner makes in deciding who should be involved in preparing the effort and whose support is needed to put it into action. Table 1–1 depicts two alternative strategies.

The selection of one strategy over another depends on the planning "climate" in the facility. If administration is generally supportive of planning and values participative management, then Strategy A may prove the more successful. On the other hand, if management tends to prefer prescriptive change rather than developmental change, Strategy B is likely to be the better approach. However, other factors also can affect the choice of strategy. For example, if the institution is in a community recently devastated by a storm, or if it or another facility were recently evaluated because of a fire, the planning climate may change. The main consideration in choosing a strategy is whether or not it is doable.

Table 1–1 Disaster Planning Strategies

Strategy considerations	Strategy A	Strategy B
Involvement	Involve people from every department in preparing the disaster plan	Involve a few people from key departments in preparing the disaster plan
Use of planning professionals	Use them for consultation only	Employ them to prepare technical parts of the plan
Completion of the plan	Allow those involved to set their own work pace	Rely on administration to set completion dates
Publicity	Maximize publicity inside and outside the facility	Minimize publicity
Planning of format	Prepare miniplan manuals tailored to individual departments	Prepare a comprehensive manual for the entire facility, with subsections for each department
Goal and objective setting	Determined by those involved in the planning	Determined by administration but with assistance of planning professionals
Cost considerations	Relatively more expensive: more personnel time devoted to meetings of the planning committee	Less expensive: fewer persons involved in meetings, but may have to hire outside experts and planning professionals
Time considerations	Generally, several months	Within weeks, if done by a planning professional

Numerous factors affect an organization's readiness for disaster planning. Exhibit 1–1 lists ten indicators and questions to ask in assessing readiness.

In an organization in which most of the indicators are affirmative, the planner probably can feel comfortable in selecting Strategy A rather than B. It is difficult to generalize, but successful disaster planning is sensitive to the experience of the people who will use the plan.

PLANNING MODELS

There are many models for planning. They range from incremental, stressing short-range planning, to long-range, comprehensive models. Figure 1–2 depicts the continuum.

Exhibit 1–1 Ten Indicators of Facility Readiness for Disaster Planning

Indicator	Key Questions	Yes	No
1. Attitudes toward planning	Is administration usually supportive of planning?	_____	_____
2. Psychology of disaster preparedness	Do few people seem frightened by the prospects of disaster?	_____	_____
3. Planning sophistication	Have many persons (clinical, administrative) had prior experience in disaster planning?	_____	_____
4. Collaboration	Is there little obvious, harmful competition between departments or units?	_____	_____
5. Decision making	Do administrators usually support decision recommendations made by subordinates?	_____	_____
6. Committees	Do most standing and ad hoc committees and task force groups complete their work thoroughly?	_____	_____
7. Prior disaster experience (internal)	Has the facility experienced some sort of internal disaster in the last three to four years (e.g., fire, earthquake)?	_____	_____
8. Prior disaster experience (external)	Has the facility responded to a casualty–generating disaster in the last three to four years?	_____	_____
9. Prior experience with disaster training	Were facility responses to disaster drills in the last three to four years satisfactory?	_____	_____
10. Stability of personnel	Are personnel turnover rates above 20 percent in the past year? If yes, in which departments or units?	_____	_____

Figure 1–2 Planning Model Continuum

Incrementalist Model — Prescriptive Model — Comprehensive Model

Charles Lindblom introduced the concept of "disjointed incrementalism" in the late 1950s.[4,5] His pioneering work suggested that decision makers (planners are decision makers) have two alternatives:

1. They can plan in comprehensive terms by identifying goals, methods, resources, and needs before beginning any action.
2. They can assume that there is no one best way to reach a goal, that obstacles will crop up, and that to be effective, plans will need to be modified.

Lindblom called the first (comprehensive) form the "root" method and suggested that, although it is useful in the scientific arena where variables are identified more easily, it is not as useful in the organizational environment. For example, in organizations, decision makers constantly encounter unexpected obstacles ranging from special interests to difficulty in gaining a consensus on goals and methods. He said that it therefore may be futile to resist this reality and that decision makers instead should embrace it. Lindblom thus called for incrementalism or, as he put it, the "branch" method of planning in organizations.

Figure 1–3 depicts the incrementalist model. Rather than beginning at a specific point in time and seeking a specific end target, the incrementalist recognizes that barriers occur, and builds flexibility into the planning process accordingly. Incrementalism assumes that there is no single, best way to achieve a goal. Instead of ignoring or trying to force events, the planner should incorporate anticipated barriers into the plan process, modifying it to cope with, overcome or, as necessary, retreat from the original path. Doing so is not interpreted as failure but rather as a response to the complexity of the organizational environment.

The comprehensive model, on the other hand, assumes that there is an agreement about goal and methods, the ability to identify and control intervening variables, and sufficient resources to reach the goal in a reasonable period of time.

Differences between the root and branch methods of planning are illustrated in the way in which discharge planners anticipate the needs of an elderly patient

Figure 1–3 Incremental Planning Process

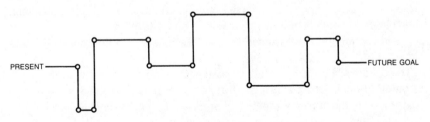

○ = Encounter with an obstacle; the plan is modified.

Exhibit 1–2 Example of Branch vs. Root Alternatives to Discharge Planning

Patient at Discharge: Caucasian male, age 74, to be discharged following abdominal surgery and three weeks' convalescence; lives with invalid wife in second–floor apartment two miles from hospital.

BRANCH ALTERNATIVE (Incremental) PLAN	ROOT ALTERNATIVE (Comprehensive) PLAN
Steps:	Steps:
1. Arrange for a visiting nurse to make an initial evaluation visit to the patient's home.	1. Arrange for visiting nurse visits daily for the first 20 days after discharge from the facility.
2. Schedule Occupational Therapy (OT), Physical Therapy (PT), and other care as identified by the visiting nurse during the initial home visit.	2. Schedule "friendly visitor" care.
	3. Schedule homemaker chore care for the first 20 days.
	4. Schedule 6 PT and 6 OT visits.
	5. Schedule transportation.
	6. Arrange for legal guardian consult.
	7. Arrange for psychiatric consult.

(Exhibit 1–2). In this case, the incremental model does not plan beyond a visit by the nurse to evaluate the home environment and problems the patient will encounter there. The assumption is that further planning will take place after the visit and that events will alter plans, so planning is short range. The comprehensive model goes much further. It defines a long list of actions that may or may not be appropriate under the circumstances; it leaves little to chance and supposes the right events will occur if they are anticipated and prescribed.

The alternative to either the incremental or the comprehensive model is the prescriptive model. Prescriptive models are used frequently in disaster planning, although they should be used with caution. Two types of prescriptive techniques are used commonly: (1) Assumed Problem Technique, (2) Off-the-Shelf Technique.[6]

The Assumed Problem Technique assumes a problem, given available data. Little additional data-gathering effort is made. The solution is assumed as obvious, as is the apparent problem. For example, a convalescent hospital was plagued with mice and cockroaches in the food service areas and on patient floors. The assumed problem was infestation, and the solution planned was facilitywide fumigation. Patient inconvenience and unpleasant publicity were anticipated outcomes, but what the planners did not expect was that infestation would continue and even increase within weeks after the plan was implemented. The wrong problem had been assumed and the wrong action taken.

The problem actually was caused by personnel negligence resulting from high turnover and inadequate training in sanitation practices. Assumed problem planning is risky. As often as not, the assumed problem is only one aspect of a situation. Therefore, actions taken may be inappropriate, costly, inconvenient, and sometimes dangerous to patient care.

The Off-the-Shelf Technique is exactly that: a prescriptive plan developed earlier. This approach is commonplace in planning. Disaster planning is no exception. Off-the-shelf plans are adopted when planners need something to present. The assumption is that because plan documents have commonalities that are transferrable from one setting to another, all that need be done is to "fill in the blanks." The advantage to this technique is that plan documents can be generated quickly. The disadvantage is that they probably will not be applicable to the setting in which they are to be used.

Effective disaster planning combines comprehensive and incremental approaches. Comprehensive planning is needed to pinpoint an overall goal and course of action tailored to meet the particular needs of the facility. But a disaster plan is only as good as its ability to mobilize and coordinate resources efficiently. Hence, to be effective, disaster plans must be tested and modified to meet incremental changes in regulations, community and personnel needs, and technology.

WHY PLAN?

Organizations facing a turbulent environment with uncertain markets and variable resources must plan carefully to survive. Those in more placid circumstances, where the market and resources are stable and certain, have less reason to plan; indeed, they have every reason to value the status quo. If their environment remains static, they will have little motivation to plan.

For many years the health care environment in the United States was placid. The certainty of the retrospective reimbursement mechanism coupled with predictability of third party payers and government policy meant that hospitals, and to a large extent skilled nursing facilities, could "float in a pleasant sea." In this climate few gave credence to the planning ethic. Indeed, until recent years virtually none of these facilities employed marketing specialists—or any other type of planning professional, for that matter.

The health care environment began to change dramatically in the early 1980s. Turbulence replaced placidity nationwide. This turbulence could be characterized by many elements: institutions scrambling to generate revenue intensified efforts to attract doctors with patients they would admit; advertising aimed directly at the consumer; price breaks to insurance companies and other payers; and marked competition in many communities. The result has been the closing of hundreds of facilities and the growth of aggressive, market-oriented, multifacility organizations. The environment for skilled nursing facilities has changed as well, with increasing emphasis on reimbursement caps, new pressure for quality care, and a continued rise in costs. Based on current trends, there is every reason to believe that this turbulence will continue through the end of the century.

The reaction of health facilities to this environment has been a rather hurried and harried adoption of planning, elevating it to much higher status than ever before. Unfortunately, this new general interest in planning does not tend to transfer readily to disaster planning specifically. Of the many reasons for this, two are paramount: (1) disaster planning does not generate revenue or save money in as direct a manner as other types of planning do; and, perhaps more important, (2) a disaster plan, to many people, is unnecessary when no disaster is imminent. In other words, until a disaster strikes, the environment is placid. The challenge for disaster planners, therefore, is to make administrators aware that the turbulence they feel elsewhere in the institution's economic and social environment is but an instant away in its physical environment. Effective disaster planning before an event occurs is an efficient way to manage the outcome.

PLANNING IN THE FACILITY: WHERE IT FITS

Planning is inherent in any bureaucratic organization. Hospitals and SNFs, regardless of size, are bureaucracies in most respects. Health care facilities prepare a variety of formal plans: annual, five-year, strategic, facility, budget, personnel, marketing, and disaster are commonplace. Planning is the means organizations use to direct their resources and/or to rationalize decisions. Some health facilities take planning more seriously than others. They allocate significant financial and personnel resources to it. The extent to which planning is supported is a barometer of management philosophy in an organization. Planning supposes that problems can be articulated, studied, and dealt with systematically. Organizations that give little more than lip service to planning in all likelihood are managed quite differently from those that do.

Centralized planning has become a common feature in today's health care facility. Centralized planning is a procedure for assigning one person or one unit in the facility to the planning role. Generally, the person or group responsible for this role generates plans and documents at the request of administration, of which they are a part. Centralized planners primarily are experts in planning, not in specialized areas such as disaster planning. Yet they often are called upon to develop or assist in the development of disaster plans because of their expertise. The risk of using centralized planners in the disaster preparedness process is that those knowledgeable in disaster response might not be consulted. In such circumstances the plan may not be appropriate to the departments with primary responsibility for handling the emergent phase of a disaster: the Emergency Department, Surgery and Postanesthesia, Communications, Security, and Administration.

Some larger hospitals have both a centralized general planning and a centralized disaster planning function (Figure 1–4).

Because of its complexity, it is helpful to view the centralized planning function as coordinative rather than technical. The coordinator's role is to bring specialists together to prepare the nuts and bolts of all kinds of plans, including those for budget, marketing, and disaster. For this role to be effective, however, the centrally based planners also must be quite knowledgeable about planning methods (although they may not know much if anything about the content of the plans they assemble).

Decentralized planning is an alternative method. It spreads planning responsibilities throughout the facility, involving many persons in the process, development, and implementation. The major benefit of decentralization is the likelihood that a plan so developed actually will be used; i.e., because people in an entity such as the Emergency Department are involved in developing their own disaster plan for that unit, they are assumed to be motivated to follow it. In the decentralized model, one person in the unit is responsible for managing its planning function.

The obvious disadvantage to decentralized planning is that it bifurcates the facility. If each department has its own plan for handling disaster, collaboration during a time of need will be a problem indeed.

Decentralized and centralized planning functions are not mutually exclusive. They should complement one another. This couples the technical aspects of centralized planning and its access to the administration of the facility with the enthusiasm of people at the unit level who ultimately must implement the plan. In this model, planning coordinators are centrally based. They assemble planning committees made up of representatives of each of the departments impacted by the plan. In some instances they organize a committee within each department, assist that group in developing its own plan, then assemble all of the plans as a facilitywide program.

The most efficient model for disaster planning uses this combined approach. A centrally based planning coordinator recruits (in collaboration with the unit supervisor) one or more planners from each unit. The unit planners hold membership on the facilitywide disaster planning committee and are responsible for data gathering pertinent to their unit. Exhibit 1–3 lists ten key questions to ask in establishing the combined planning model.

Figure 1-4 Centralized and Specialized Planning Functions in a Tertiary Care Hospital

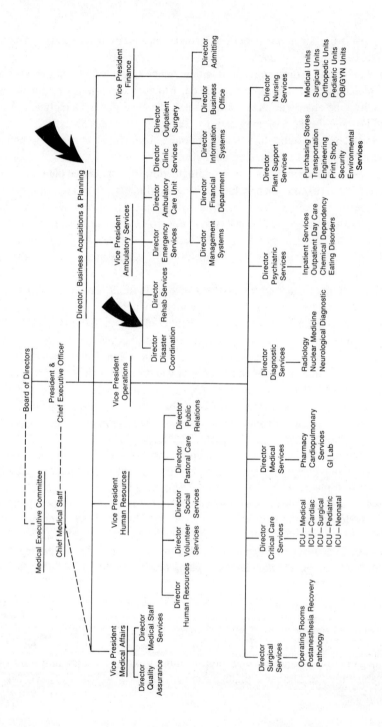

Exhibit 1–3 Action Checklist for a Combined Centralized-Decentralized
Disaster Planning Model

Ten Key Questions	*Yes*	*No*
1. Has someone been assigned the role of Disaster Planning Coordinator for the entire facility?	_____	_____
2. Is that Coordinator skilled or experienced in developing and preparing written plans?	_____	_____
3. Has an inventory been made of the disaster planning needs of each department or unit?	_____	_____
4. Has an annual master schedule of all plans needed by all departments been prepared, including the disaster plan and manual? (It should specify completion deadlines, the persons who must approve the plans, and the persons needed to complete them.)	_____	_____
5. Do department managers know how to request assistance from the Coordinator?	_____	_____
6. Do all units or departments use a standard format for making requests and listing identified needs?	_____	_____
7. Is there a procedure for evaluating the plan after it has been approved by the appropriate levels of management and for checking whether it is being followed?	_____	_____
8. Is appropriate training linked to the plan? Are people adequately trained to put it into operation?	_____	_____
9. Are unit planners trained for their role and given sufficient release time from their usual assignments to participate in planning activities?	_____	_____
10. Does the Coordinator have the financial resources to hire planning consultants and disaster specialists to assist in the planning, in preparing the disaster manual, and in training facility personnel once the plan and manual are completed?	_____	_____

WHO ARE THE PLANNERS?

Disaster planning is a serious activity that should not be delegated to an obscure level in the organization. Unfortunately, some facilities fail to accentuate the importance of disaster planning.

The Joint Commission on Accreditation of Hospitals (JCAH) requires that hospitals prepare and document the use of disaster plans. It does not specify who should be involved.

Effective disaster planners come from all walks of life and academic backgrounds, but they share important attributes which include the ability to:

1. conceptualize and to imagine alternative futures
2. take data such as census information or diagnosis related group (DRG) reports and identify patterns in the data
3. analyze a problem logically in a step-by-step manner
4. ask questions of peers, administrators, and technical specialists
5. write reports and abstract from reports
6. lead groups effectively and encourage people to contribute their ideas
7. be patient
8. admit that they do not have all of the answers themselves.

SUMMARY

Planning is rational. It assumes that it is possible for individuals to anticipate problems, control events, and "make the future happen" by organizing activities and people. Planning as a value is integral to the sciences. As such, health professionals would be expected to adopt the planning construct. Many health facilities, although giving the appearance of operating differently, did not begin to practice systematic planning until recent years. Today, virtually every acute care hospital and skilled nursing facility has a part-time or full-time person involved in some type of organizational planning. Numerous clinicians, particularly nurses, are involved now in quality assurance and discharge-planning activities.

Yet, in spite of widespread practice, disaster planning in many facilities tends to receive only modest and superficial attention. One probable reason was previously discussed that while planning assumes control leading to a certain outcome, event, or benefit, disaster planning is the act of planning for how to respond to an uncontrollable event. Because of this and because a disaster is "unthinkable," it is difficult for health professionals—people who otherwise value rationality and control—to invest in disaster planning with the same enthusiasm as they do other types of planning.

Planning strategy is the path the expert takes to "sell" planning in the facility. One type of strategy favors maximum involvement of personnel and outsiders in the planning, while another strategy sees planning as more the responsibility of professionals.

Some planners favor incremental, others prescriptive, and still others comprehensive planning models. Each has advantages and disadvantages.

The planning function in some facilities is centralized, in others decentralized. For disaster planning, a combination of the two is recommended. Planning can be learned, but it requires core abilities, including the ability to organize and manage a diverse group of individuals.

NOTES

1. Weston H. Agor, *Intuitive Management: Integrating Left and Right Brain Management Skills.* (Englewood Cliffs, NJ: Prentice-Hall, 1984), 1–7.

2. Sid Segalowitz, *The Two Sides of the Brain: Brain Lateralization Explored.* (Englewood Cliffs, NJ: Prentice-Hall, 1983), 94.

3. Genesis 1:28.

4. Charles Lindblom, "The Science of Muddling Through." *Public Administration Review* 19 (Spring 1959): 77–88.

5. _____, "Still Muddling, Not Yet Through." *Public Administration Review* 36 (November/December 1979): 517–24.

6. Paul Nutt, *Planning Methods for Health and Related Organizations.* (New York: John Wiley & Sons, 1984), 72–84.

REFERENCES

Azarnoff, Roy, and Seliger, Jerome. *Delivering Human Services.* Englewood Cliffs, NJ: Prentice-Hall, Inc., 1982, 10–122.

De Bono, Edward. *Lateral Thinking: Creativity by Step.* New York: Harper & Row, 1970.

Deutsch, George, and Springer, Sally. *Left Brain, Right Brain.* San Francisco: W.H. Freeman, 1981.

Havelock, R.G. *Planning for Innovation.* Ann Arbor, MI: Center for Utilization of Scientific Knowledge, 1973.

Kallman, Ernest, Reinharth, Leon, and Shapiro, H. Jack. *The Practice of Planning—Strategic Administrative and Operational.* New York: Van Nostrand Reinhold, 1981.

Rodgers, E.M. *The Diffusion of Innovation.* New York: The Free Press, 1962.

Chapter 2

The Planning Process

Planning is a developmental, rational process for solving problems. The more complex the problem, the greater the need for systematizing, or formulating, an approach to solving it. The problem-solving process for purposes here involves seven distinct steps and associated activities.

The seven-step process is important for two reasons:

1. It is a systematic way of developing a plan.
2. It is used frequently as the format for compiling a written plan.

In this chapter the seven steps are prescribed as the sequence that disaster planners should use in developing a plan document.

STEP 1: PROBLEM SENSING

The ability to "feel" or sense a problem is vital to the problem-solving process both in everyday life and in an organization. Just as nerves in the skin warn when a hot object is touched, problem–sensing activities point to changing needs and conditions. Accurate and early sensing, whether intuitive or the result of some sort of managerial feedback process in an organization, signals a warning of problems.

Problem sensing precedes planning and is the step that highlights problems for further analysis. Once a problem is sensed and its indicators are stated in writing, planning can begin.

The more descriptive the written problem statement, the easier it will be to develop the steps in the planning process. Many organizations so respect this sensing role that they have institutionalized it by hiring systems analysts, action researchers, and program planners whose job is to identify problems as early as possible and feed their findings to management for appropriate action.

Identifying problem indicators is difficult. The following cases are illustrative.

Problem–Sensing Case # 1

The Fire Marshal made headlines recently by citing the city's own large, infant and child board-and-care facility (300 beds) for crowding, inadequate and blocked exits, and uncovered combustibles. This was not the first such news story. A young physician completing a residency in pediatrics at the facility described a host of problems to a TV reporter. The physician recalled a fire drill in which a cottage dormitory with 30 children was "overlooked and forgotten " in the drill. She also said that the majority of infants and toddlers in the nursery had low fevers, body rashes that did not seem to respond to usual treatment, elevated pulse rates, shallow respiration, and constipation. Staff members seemed ill equipped to handle things. Their usual approach was to give the quiet babies a bottle and look after the noisier ones.

Problem Indicators

This case suggests several problems, any one or all may be used to develop a plan for action. Possible problem areas include:

- Fire Code violations and disaster preparedness
- inadequate personnel supervision
- inadequate clinical treatment
- inadequate personnel training
- children seriously stressed.

Problem–Sensing Case # 2

The fire in the McLeod Apartments in January was the third in less than three months. Unlike the previous fires, this one apparently began in the electrical wiring inside an elevator control cab. Twenty casualties were taken to the local Emergency Department in shock or obvious trauma; many had burns and smoke inhalation. At the time of their arrival the emergency physician was the only doctor on duty in the hospital. Triage was delayed for 45 minutes after arrival of the first victim because of insufficient personnel to perform the function. In addition, victims arrived untagged, with minimal field assessment and incorrect triage priorities. The hospital had received inadequate prior warning with insufficient information about the incident.

Problem Indicators

This case presents several problems, any or all of which could be used as a basis for revising existing facility and community disaster plans:

- probable inadequate preventative fire inspection
- lack of landlord compliance with fire and building codes
- inconsistent triage procedures by field personnel
- insufficient number of hospital triage personnel on duty or acquired
- inadequate hospital callback procedures
- inadequate advance notification to the hospital.

One technique helpful in systematically sensing for problems is illustrated by how the disaster coordinator of a 160-bed acute care hospital in New Jersey handles the role. Two short (30 to 45 minutes) meetings are held annually with all department heads or their designees. The purpose of the meetings is to recall, then brainstorm, major change events affecting the hospital in the preceding six months.

The meeting is begun by the disaster coordinator who asks about service, staffing, and facility changes. The coordinator then requests participants to recall any changes in public transportation, public safety, and other events in the hospital's service area, using a large flip chart to record responses quickly and in full view of the participants. (Typical responses are presented in Exhibit 2–1.) The meetings become livelier and more relaxed as events are recalled. The disaster coordinator, who not incidentally has excellent group process skills, facilitates the meeting and encourages ideas.

Exhibit 2–1 Example of Brainstormed Ideas from a Problem-Sensing Meeting

What has occurred at Hospital X since last November?

- Joe A. has been replaced as head of Housekeeping.
- A PPO is contracting with us. This will mean more patients for the outpatient wing.
- Rumors say the hospital may be designated as a trauma center by the county.
- The Smith Street side of the building will be remodeled next month.
- A layoff of about 20 percent of RNs, PTs, RPTs can be expected because of DRGs.
- Mary S. had a baby.
- Hotel fire survivors were treated quickly by the ED (we got great publicity, too).

This technique has been in use for three years and has become a popular activity. Participants look forward to it in the same way they do to a going-away party. It is a nonthreatening opportunity to share "memories" with a congenial group of peers.

As Exhibit 2–1 suggests, several indicators with implications for disaster planning emerged from this problem-sensing group experience:

- The new head of a major service unit (Housekeeping) will need orientation and training in the use of the disaster plan.
- Closure of an entrance to the facility will require temporary revision of evacuation segments of the plan.
- The trauma center rumor, if true, may mean comprehensive revision of the disaster plan.
- Personnel layoffs have the potential for disrupting callback procedures in the plan and create a need for disaster preparedness training of any new hires.
- Mary S.'s absence for three months necessitates designating someone to take over her PBX role.

The same group problem-sensing technique can be used with representatives of health facilities, public safety agencies, and so forth. Group problem sensing has a clear advantage over other survey techniques such as telephone, mail, and interviews with individuals. It not only can be fun, because people enjoy getting together and brainstorming, it also can provide a wealth of information when individual responses produce recall and stimulate others to contribute ideas as well.

In addition to activities such as group sensing, other sources for sensing data include:

- secondary data from census reports, public health morbidity and mortality statistics, and facility census reports
- interviews with providers, vendors, and consumers
- the planner's own intuitive feelings
- observation of personnel and volunteer response to actual disaster events or disaster drills.

Whether the issues sensed are important ultimately depends on further analysis and decisions by planners and plan sponsors, such as the facility's administration.

STEP 2: GOAL SETTING

The second step in the planning process is to define clear goals for the plan. Goals are statements that broadly depict desired futures. They provide targets for action and constitute a justification for action. Goals also serve as standards for gauging an organization's effectiveness and efficiency. As such, they are used to evaluate whether or not an action has achieved what was intended.[1]

Objectives are subordinate to goals. They specify milestones that must be met in order to reach the goal. Objectives should not be defined until the problem has been analyzed thoughtfully, i.e., until after steps three and four of the problem-solving process have been completed.

Disaster plans may require more than one goal. Typical goals in disaster plans include:

- rapid admission and treatment of casualties
- initial and continued medical care for casualties and seriously ill non-casualties
- protection of evacuated patients as required.

These general statements are useful and easily incorporated into a plan. Unfortunately, many planners are too quick to adopt what others have developed as goals because, to quote a director of nursing at a disaster preparedness seminar, "Everyone knows what a disaster plan is." That may or may not be true, but what is certain is that goal statements that are more specific to the institution are much more useful than general statements.

Goal statements must be clear and unambiguous. The following are examples:

1. The goal of the Crenshaw Convalescent Home is to provide chronic care to medically indigent adults in North County.
2. Our goal for 1990 is outreach to 1,100 high-risk consumers and to reduce deaths from trauma below 1985–1990 rates.
3. The goal of the Tri-County Community Hospital Disaster Plan is to provide medical treatment to all incoming casualties with a minimum time delay.

It is helpful to specify a target population in a goal statement, as in example 1. If applicable, the goals also should be quantified, as in example 2. The latter not only targets a population and a category of action—"high-risk"—but it also specifies a performance standard—"below 1985–1990 rates." These, plus goal 3, are ways to express goals for a disaster plan, but although they identify a target population and a category of action, the statements are not quantifiable. Example 3 can be modified to do so: "The goal of the Tri-County Community Hospital Disaster Plan is to provide medical treatment to a minimum of 10 major and 50 minor casualties within five minutes of their receipt."

The final approval authority for disaster plan goals is very important. Without the backing of the facility's administration it is uncertain whether the planning process and the plan per se will be followed. For example, unless the hospital's chief executive officer (CEO) sees disaster planning as a meaningful activity it will be difficult to get personnel assigned to its development and writing or to participate in drills. If administration does not support the disaster plan concept when goals are established, it is not likely to do so enthusiastically later on.

Involving policymakers will reinforce the importance of the plan. The goals also should reflect consensus on the part of the facility's board and/or senior managers. One technique for gaining consensus from this group is for the disaster planner to prepare draft versions of the goal(s) in memo form, including a background statement describing how the goals were developed and what they will be used for (Exhibit 2–2).

Depending on how the facility is managed, the memo should be presented to policymakers (in this example, to the executive committee of the board) for consideration and a decision. The planner should attend the meetings to provide technical consultation as requested.

STEP 3: NEEDS ASSESSMENT

This step in the planning process is important for two reasons: (1) It is the method for carefully examining the problem at which the plan is aimed, and (2) it

---

Exhibit 2–2 Example of Goal Statement Approval Memo

6/12/88
TO: Executive Committee, AC Hospital
FROM: R.J.S., Disaster Planning Coordinator
SUBJECT: Disaster Plan Goals

Background

JCAH will visit the hospital next March. In anticipation, we are revising our Disaster Plan. In order to begin we must have clear goals in mind. Two goals are proposed. Please consider them carefully and make any modifications that you feel are needed. Attached is a copy of the JCAH requirements as well as a critique by the Disaster Planning Committee of our current Disaster Plan goals.

Goal # 1: In the event of an external disaster, AC Hospital will be able to provide rapid and efficient medical care to incoming casualties.

Goal # 2: In the event of a facility overload, AC Hospital will be able to evacuate 30 medical plaza patients safely within 15 minutes of notification.

MODIFICATIONS:

is an excellent mechanism for involving others. The planner determines the scope of the problem by performing a needs assessment.

The manner in which needs assessment findings are reported in plan documents varies. Some documents contain a section titled "Background," others use "Problem Description," still others use "Need." That last item is the most descriptive word for a disaster plan and thus is used here. Descriptions of need can be stated in narrative form, in quantitative terms, or in a combination of the types. There are advantages and disadvantages for each, although the combined use of narrative, descriptive, and quantitative information probably is most useful because they reinforce one another (Table 2–1).

A major task to be handled cautiously in writing a needs statement is to limit the amount of information while providing enough to understand the problem more clearly. Too much information can be overwhelming; conversely, too little will be of no use. Possibly the best method to use in determining needs is to assemble persons with experience to brainstorm the scope of need. The questions to be asked will differ from facility to facility. For example, if the goal is to ready a skilled nursing facility to handle an internal disaster, the questions to be asked will be quite different from those if the goal is to prepare a mental health clinic to handle victims from a hallucinogen party. The following are key questions for developing a disaster planning needs assessment:

Table 2–1 Examples of Needs Descriptions: Paramedic Retrieval Time for Various Locations in a Disaster

Narrative Form of Needs Description	Quantitative Form of Needs Description		
Fully two-thirds of the community's acute care beds are occupied all of the time. On the average, retrieval time of paramedic ambulances from the airport will range from 8 to 11 minutes, depending on time of day. The nearest level-one trauma facility is nearly 30 minutes away during peak traffic periods. Response times, retrieval times, and bed status during a disaster will affect our ability to handle a large number of casualties.	Facility	Disaster Site	Average Retrieval Time (Minutes)
	G.H. Hospital	Downtown	13
		Airport	11
		S. Town	6
	University Medical Center	Downtown	3
		Airport	30
		S. Town	24
	R. Hospital	Downtown	18
		Airport	37
		S. Town	3

1. How many beds does the facility have?
2. What is the daily average occupancy?
3. How many staff members are on duty each shift?
4. How often does the facility have a disaster drill?
5. Is the disaster plan current for both internal and external incidents?
6. What type and number of health services and public safety agencies are within five miles of the facility?
7. What are the current demographics of the facility's service area (census, morbidity, mortality data)?
8. What emergency communication links are currently available and operational in the facility? With whom are the links?
9. What potential disaster sites are within 10, 25, 50 miles of the facility (e.g., airports, petrochemical plants, etc.)?
10. Who within the facility has received and maintained certificates or licenses related to disaster response capability (cardiopulmonary resuscitation [CPR], Advanced Cardiac Life Support provider, emergency/trauma care)?
11. What large community events can be expected (e.g., rock concerts, parades) that may generate casualties in the event of a disaster?
12. What is the weather like in this community (e.g., are tornadoes, hurricanes, floods episodic; if so, at what times during the year)?

Once the questions have been asked, the next step is to gather the data. Several of the techniques for doing so are listed in Figure 2–1 and described next. The technique chosen depends upon the interest and resources of the planner.

The problem in needs assessment is to know what is really important and what questions to ask. The data-gathering techniques in Figure 2–1 can be used in two ways: (1) as a means for finding out what questions to ask before actual data gathering begins, and (2) as a means for gathering data in order to prepare the needs statement.

Literature—Secondary Sources Technique

This involves examining existing secondary data sources such as census information, other public records, facility records, facility plans, and the professional and academic literature. Sources can include the institution's library, public and university libraries, public and comprehensive health planning jurisdictions such as health systems agencies, regional planning jurisdictions, and the federal government.

Brainstorming Technique

Brainstorming is the easiest and most popular technique. Here, the convenor brings together a group of experts and brainstorms them for ideas. Questions are

Figure 2–1 Needs Assessment Steps

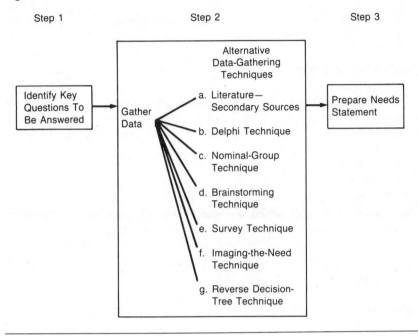

asked, quick responses are encouraged, and criticism of responses is discouraged. Responses are listed on a flip chart or blackboard. The group then can be brainstormed again to place the responses in priority, to decide what should be done with the list, etc. Brainstorming is a practical technique that puts people at ease and encourages participation.

The Delphi Technique

In this method (named for the mythological Greek oracle of Delphi), the judgments of knowledgeable people are collated and synthesized. The planner gathers a group of experts who have knowledge of disaster planning and response: specialists from the fire department, chemists experienced with combustibles, explosives experts from the military or police, mental health specialists, planners from other facilities, and so forth.

Assembling the group in the same room will save time, although this is not mandatory for the technique to work. If members are together, the planner in charge of the meeting instructs them not to talk with one another once the Delphi activity begins. Each member is given the same question and is asked to write a response on a notepad. The responses are gathered and recorded. The members are asked next to respond to the list of responses. The cycle is repeated until the convenor feels there is sufficient consensus among the experts, i.e., about the ideas generated, their importance, etc.[2]

This technique is an excellent way to identify the questions that need answering in order to develop the needs assessment.

Nominal Group Technique

In this technique, a panel of experts is brought together in the same room at the same time. Instead of asking first for ideas, the group's convenor (usually the planner) poses a key question or issue, such as "What should be examined, given the problem and goal stated in our disaster plan?"

The process then is as follows:

1. Members respond in writing without talking.
2. The convenor, after gathering responses, verbally brainstorms the group to recall their written responses. These are written on a flip chart or blackboard.
3. The convenor then involves the group in an oral critique of each idea.
4. The group, after a discussion of the pros and cons of each idea, votes to list the ideas by priority.[3]

Survey Technique

There are seven types of surveys useful for both identifying questions to ask about needs and for determining needs.

1. personal interview
2. telephone interview
3. group interview
4. mail questionnaire
5. encounter interview
6. drive-by or "windshield" survey (impressions of a situation or setting as the planner drives through the community)
7. literature, secondary document search.

As with the needs assessment techniques discussed previously, the first step is to determine the purpose of the survey: What does the planner want to know? The next step is to determine who has the information. Exhibit 2–3 presents a decision checklist useful in preparing a survey to gather information.

The fundamental purpose of a needs assessment is to generate baseline information. In disaster planning, the planners or their designees generally seek out expert input for baseline information. Personal interviews or mailed questionnaires can be the most expeditious way to obtain information from this type of group. The

Exhibit 2–3 Needs Assessment Survey Decision Checklist

	Yes	No
1. Is the purpose of this survey clear?	____	____
2. Do you want information from specific persons rather than individuals selected at random?	____	____
3. Are personal interviews necessary?	____	____
4. Are group interviews necessary?	____	____
5. Can questionnaires be distributed by mail?	____	____
6. Can questionnaires devised for other needs surveys be used in this survey?	____	____
7. Will you design the questionnaire yourself?	____	____
8. Will you design the methodology for carrying out the survey yourself?	____	____
9. Will the questionnaires use closed–ended questions?	____	____
10. Will the questionnaires use open–ended questions?	____	____
11. Will the questionnaire be designed for easy computer coding and input?	____	____
12. Do you have the personal and personnel resources to carry out the survey?	____	____

advantage of using a questionnaire is that it can force the respondents, depending on whether the document uses open- or closed-ended questions and how they are phrased, to react to specific points, issues, or problems. Exhibit 2–4 lists examples of closed- and open-ended questions.

If a questionnaire is mailed, state the reasons for asking the questions and provide an explanation of how the data will be analyzed. Questions should be short and as unambiguous as possible. The entire questionnaire should be as brief as possible but should include explanatory material to help focus the responses.

The disadvantage of a mailed questionnaire is that respondents do not have an opportunity to discuss it or interact with the interviewer, and vice versa. In a mailed survey, it is not unusual for 50 percent or more of the recipients not to return the questionnaire unless it is preceded by personal or telephone contact.

Imaging–the–Need Technique

In this technique, the planner or planning coordinator assembles the group in one room. Participants can be expert or not. The technique works best, however, if

Exhibit 2–4 Examples of Closed- and Open-Ended Questions in a Needs
Assessment Questionnaire with Expert Respondents

Closed-Ended Examples

1. What triage classification is in use in the hospital?
   - a. five-tiered
   - b. four-tiered
   - c. three-tiered
   - d. two-tiered

2. How many patients would an explosion at the paper mill generate if the explosion occurs during peak work hours?
   - a. under 10
   - b. 10–15
   - c. 15–20
   - d. 25–30
   - e. more than 30

3. Which neighborhoods are at most risk from flood damage?
   - a. Fremont
   - b. Alta Loma
   - c. Marystown
   - d. Manchester
   - e. Garfield

Open-Ended Examples

1. If casualties will be coming from the northwest, what is the best way to control the flow of vehicular traffic at our Broadway Street entrances? (Maps of site and streets are attached.)

   _____

   _____

2. How can we address the fears of our personnel about family survival in the event of a serious earthquake?

   _____

   _____

---

they are familiar with the facility and its routines. Imaging the need involves three steps:

1. The planner, acting as facilitator, asks the group members to close their eyes and imagine the facility's responding to an external disaster, then asks, "What do you 'see' with your eyes closed?" Individuals call out their responses, which are recorded on a flip chart: "Confusion," "Shocked," "Out of it," "Excitement," "A problem with Joe in the guard shack," "Everyone running," etc.

2. The facilitator asks the group to think about an internal disaster in the facility, then repeats the "What do you 'see' . . .?" question.
3. The facilitator lists the responses on the flip chart, then brainstorms needs. The facilitator points to the internal and external lists and says: "Look at these adjectives" (excited, confused, shocked). "Why do you think so? Why do you feel as you do? What needs do the statements indicate?" The facilitator lists these needs on another flip chart. The process is repeated until all of the words or ideas imaged are discussed.

Imaging the need is fun. Individuals have a good time sharing what they "see" and are comfortable participating. It is not only a means of identifying personnel training needs in a nonthreatening manner, it is also an excellent means for identifying planning needs.

Reverse Decision-Tree Technique

A technique for determining tasks necessary to achieve a goal and objectives is the decision tree.* The sequence of steps for developing a decision tree is as follows.

1. Identify a specific goal (future).
2. Identify objectives necessary to reach the stated goal.
3. Identify major tasks to accomplish each of the objectives.
4. List the tasks by priority.

The decision tree is an extremely useful needs assessment tool. It specifies what must be accomplished in order to reach the goal. The entire project is expedited because the process that must be followed is identified clearly. Decision trees help group members visualize their ideas and the process of developing the tree stimulates brainstorming and decision. Figure 2–2 is an example of the technique applied to an earthquake needs assessment.

To develop a reverse decision tree, a group of experts (or others) is assembled in a conference room. If goals have been determined previously and approved (by the facility's board of directors, for instance), these are written on a flip chart or otherwise posted in a prominent place in the room. If goals have not been determined, the facilitator brainstorms the group for goals and writes them on the flip chart.

---

*Just as a living tree has a trunk, limbs, and branches, the decision tree branches in different directions pointing the decision maker away from the "trunk," i.e., the goal statement, and toward different paths.

Figure 2–2 Example of Decision-Tree Needs Assessment Technique (As Used with a Group to Identify Earthquake-Related Needs)

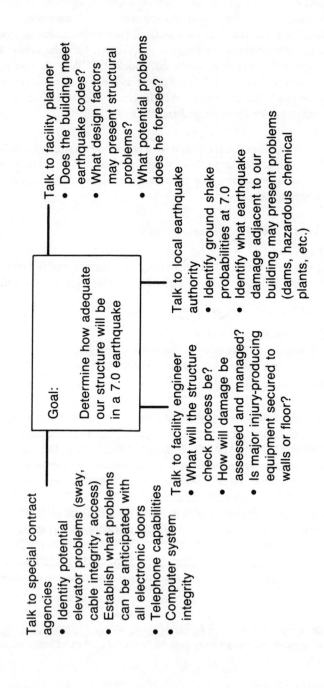

Goal:

Determine how adequate our structure will be in a 7.0 earthquake

Talk to special contract agencies
• Identify potential elevator problems (sway, cable integrity, access)
• Establish what problems can be anticipated with all electronic doors
• Telephone capabilities
• Computer system integrity

Talk to facility engineer
• What will the structure check process be?
• How will damage be assessed and managed?
• Is major injury-producing equipment secured to walls or floor?

Talk to facility planner
• Does the building meet earthquake codes?
• What design factors may present structural problems?
• What potential problems does he foresee?

Talk to local earthquake authority
• Identify ground shake probabilities at 7.0
• Identify what earthquake damage adjacent to our building may present problems (dams, hazardous chemical plants, etc.)

Using inductive reasoning, the facilitator asks the participants to "think backward" from the goal and identify objectives needed to meet it, then lists them on the flip chart (see Figure 2–2, above). The facilitator next brainstorms the group for ways to categorize the objectives and lists them in clockwise fashion around each goal statement. The group is brainstormed again for tasks needed to implement the objectives.

Once needs have been determined, the planner's role is to compare the data with stated goal(s), then develop a needs assessment statement. The statement usually is prepared in narrative form, with backup statistics and other references appended. The needs assessment should be straightforward and descriptive, noting as many of the relevant facts as possible without overwhelming the reader with detail. Exhibit 2–5 is an excerpt from a needs statement based upon the decision-tree data cited earlier.

Exhibit 2–5 Excerpt from a Needs Assessment Statement

On March 7, 19___, the planning group determined that General Hospital must assess the structural adequacy of its tower and main building in the event of an earthquake of 7.0 magnitude. Upon investigating, we discovered the following:

1. Our buildings meet earthquake codes for the state in their general construction.
2. Ground shake of 7.0 beneath our facility will produce the following ground results:

   a. The natural mixture of sandy loam and shale beneath the west wing is likely to lead to the collapse of the annex housing ambulatory psychiatric patients.
   b. The intake drive for rescue vehicles is likely to become obstructed by debris from the eucalyptus tree at the entrance.
   c. The overhead canopy across the driveway into the parking area will collapse unless reinforced.

3. Major equipment items in the laboratory, all unit clean utility rooms, and physical therapy must be bolted to walls and/or floor.
4. Machines in the laundry room are not on flex cables and may pull free from the walls if the ground shifts beneath them.
5. Computer patient records retrieval will be unavailable, requiring a backup manual system. It also is conceivable that all records may be lost.
6. Elevator cabs are designed to permit only limited vertical slippage in a 7.0 earthquake. Expected lateral sway would be approximately 30°. Stress on the cable is likely to result in car drop of not more than 1 to 2 feet. Expected injuries in cabs will depend on number of passengers, degree of sway, and degree of drop. Planning must be based on a "worst case" scenario.

STEP 4: OBJECTIVE SETTING

This step in the planning process involves specifying what action is to be taken and when.

An objective is a desired accomplishment or hoped-for result. It is a dimension of a goal that has a narrower focus and a shorter time frame than a goal. Insofar as possible, objectives should be expressed as quantitative, or otherwise measurable, time-specific statements.

There are many ways to state objectives. Three examples are detailed next. Once a format for writing objectives is decided upon, it should be used consistently to lessen ambiguity and to aid in evaluating whether the plan succeeds or fails.

Example 1: As a result of changes in referral patterns during the 1988–89 program year, patient processing will be increased to three per hour.

Example 2: Referrals from the reception area to the rehabilitation center will increase by 8 percent over 1988 levels in the 1989 program year.

Example 3: Inservice education will teach disaster preparedness to at least 100 clinical staff members, commencing in 1990 and continuing annually.

Example 1 assumes that action will have taken place, as suggested by the words "As a result of . . . ;" Example 2 is a directive for action (i.e., "will increase . . ."). Both forms have the attributes of specifying what will happen and when and of quantifying outcomes. Example 3, however, is preferred by most planners because the objective is stated in discrete increments, making it easier to assess later whether the objective has been met. When selecting a format, it should be kept in mind that an objective is a written statement of a desired accomplishment or hoped-for result. It is only one dimension of the goal. As much as possible, an objective should be written in quantitative, measurable, concrete terms.[4]

Certain verbs and phrases are not useful in preparing written objectives because they are difficult to quantify:

appreciate   know
believe   listen
comprehend   perceive
experience   think
feel   understand

Table 2–2 Verbs Frequently Used in Preparing Plan Objectives

Activities	Analysis	Tasks	Action
attempt	analyze	articulate	act
attend	appraise	assemble	choose
complete	categorize	bend	clasp
copy	compare	build	communicate
count	deduce	capitalize	cooperate
indicate	discover	classify	demonstrate
isolate	evaluate	compound	display
label	expand	construct	distinguish
list	formulate	coordinate	grasp
locate	generalize	count	inform
map	generate	depict	interact
order	identify	dissect	participate
organize	induce	drop	place
record	infer	estimate	reduce
repeat	modify	graph	relate
reproduce	plan	handle	reset
select	predict	illustrate	separate
state	present	increase	serve
tally	propose	make	specify
	question	measure	transfer
	restructure	plot	weigh
	simplify	reduce	
	structure	rewrite	
	summarize	solve	
	synthesize	summarize	
		tabulate	
		verbalize	
		verify	
		write	

Table 2–2 lists verbs that would be useful in preparing objectives.[5]
Regardless of which form is used, objectives must be:

1. within the authority of the facility
2. within the range of competence of the institution in terms of its organization, personnel, equipment, and facilities
3. feasible within budget limits
4. legal
5. compatible with the moral and value judgment of those affected by the objective
6. practical and capable of being implemented
7. unencumbered by unpleasant side effects
8. acceptable to those expected to carry them out
9. measurable.[6]

STEP 5: ACTION PLAN DETAILING

This step specifies how the objectives will be met, what activities will be needed to achieve them, who will be responsible for each activity, and when each will be completed. The decision-tree technique can be used initially to determine activities, although a detailed action plan should be developed and distributed to all of those involved.

Action plan detailing is analogous to a blueprint. It gives direction to everyone involved in plan implementation. This blueprint for action may include tables and charts detailing the who-what/who-when, and can be quite extensive. Action plan details should be incorporated into the facility's disaster manual. Some disaster manuals are virtually all tables and charts prescribing activities and assigning responsibility for action. Others contain more narrative as well as some detailing. Figure 2–3 outlines the sequence for developing an action plan detailing.

1. Scope-of-Work Chart

The first step in detailing is to develop a Scope-of-Work Chart. The chart contains five components:

1. goal statement
2. objective(s) statement
3. implementation activities
4. timeline
5. methods for evaluating outcomes.

Exhibit 2–6 illustrates use of the Scope-of-Work Chart format. The example used is for a disaster preparedness training program to ready providers to assist homebound disabled persons following a disaster. The Scope-of-Work Chart must

Figure 2–3 Sequence for Development of Action Plan Detail

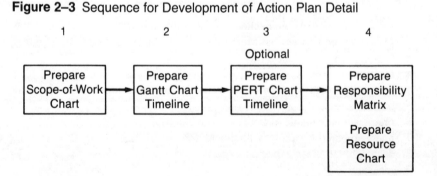

Exhibit 2–6 Example of Scope-of-Work Chart

Goal: Increase the disaster response capabilities of Maxwell County chronic care providers to serve the estimated 300 at-risk elderly persons in the Sun Valley River basin.

Objective	Implementation Action	Time	Method to Evaluate
1. As a result of participation in a training workshop, 40 chronic care personnel will be able to identify the service needs of eligible disabled patients who are homebound during a disaster.	1.1 The Disaster Plan staff will assemble an Advisory Committee composed of representatives of ten chronic care providers in the county, disabled support groups, and public safety agencies.	1/1/87-3/31/87	An evaluation questionnaire will be developed by the Disaster Coordinator. It will include closed- and open-ended items, and true/false items. All participants in the training workshop will complete the questionnaire so the extent to which objective # 1 has been met can be determined.
	1.2 Staff will prepare a draft curriculum for an eight-hour workshop to be held in two-hour time blocks biweekly	2/1/87-2/28/87	
	1.3 The Disaster Advisory Committee will meet monthly for first three months, then trimonthly, to: a. assess and critique the curriculum developed by the Coordinator b. identify training workshop speakers c. assess and critique evaluation instruments d. assist in publicizing the training event.	3/5/87-6/30/87	
	1.4 The Disaster Plan staff will conduct telephone survey of 30 percent of the estimated 100 chronic care personnel in the county to determine extent of their education about disasters and about the service needs of at-risk elderly persons in a disaster.	3/5/87-5/15/87	
	1.5 The staff will schedule and publicize the event.	5/15/87-6/30/87	
	1.6 The staff will conduct four two-hour training workshops at four sites throughout the county.	7/1/87-6/30/88	

be provided to everyone involved in the planning; they will refer to their own copy frequently as work progresses. While the sample shown reflects only one page of such a chart, complete charts can cover several pages.

2. Gantt Timeline Chart

A Gantt Chart is a helpful supplement to the Scope-of-Work Chart. Named after its developer in the early part of this century, industrial engineer, Henry Gantt, the method is used to depict the relationship of time to events as a simple bar chart. The Gantt Chart is used to track the progress of intended activities visually. Mounting the chart on a wall where planning committee members can refer to it readily ensures its use and helps remind everyone of task completion dates. Exhibit 2–7 is an example of a Gantt Chart covering the same activities outlined in Exhibit 2–6.

3. PERT Chart

The Gantt Chart does not reflect interactive relationships; for that purpose some planners use a PERT chart (Program Evaluation and Review Technique). PERT enables managers to foresee how program activities are linked with one another and identifies the timing of a decision and its effect. Basic to PERT is the sequencing of related events and activities into a network.

Figure 2–4 illustrates the use of PERT in planning for the renovation of a hospital open-heart surgery unit. It and the description of the PERT method are reprinted here with the permission of Reston Publishing Company, Inc.*

Events are represented by boxes in the network; activities are represented by arrows connecting events. It should be noted that some events may depend on only a single prior event while, in other situations, there may be an interrelationship of several events leading to the accomplishment of an ultimate objective. Figure 2–4 illustrates the three basic characteristics of a program or project that are amenable to the PERT approach. The first characteristic is that activities must be such that *time estimates* can be made. In the example, it is possible to estimate how long it will take to accomplish each activity. Secondly, there must be definite starting and ending points. Without them, there could be no events that are the beginning or ending of an activity. Finally, and this is the key to PERT's usefulness, there must be parallel activities. That is,

---

*From Beaufort Longest, Jr., *Management Practices for the Health Professional*, 3rd ed., 1984. Reprinted by permission of Reston Publishing Company, a Prentice-Hall Company, 11480 Sunset Hills Road, Reston, VA 22090.

Exhibit 2–7 Example of Gantt Chart

Goal: Increase the disaster response capabilities of Maxwell County chronic care providers to serve the estimated 300 at–risk homebound elderly persons in the Sun Valley River basin.

Objectives: As a result of participation in an eight–hour training workshop series, 40 chronic care personnel will be able to identify the service needs of eligible patients who are homebound during a disaster.

Implementation Activities

1.1 Advisory Committee composed of ten or more chronic care providers in the county will be assembled.

1.2 Disaster Coordinator (Plan Staff) will prepare a draft curriculum for an eight–hour training workshop to be held in two–hour time blocks biweekly.

1.3 Advisory Committee will:

    a. assess and critique curriculum

    b. identify training workshop speakers

    c. assess and critique evaluation instruments

    d. assist in publicizing the training event.

1.4 Staff will conduct a telephone survey of 30 percent of the 100 chronic care personnel in the county.

1.5 Staff will schedule and publicize the training event.

1.6 Staff will conduct four two–hour training workshops at four sites throughout the county beginning 7/1/87.

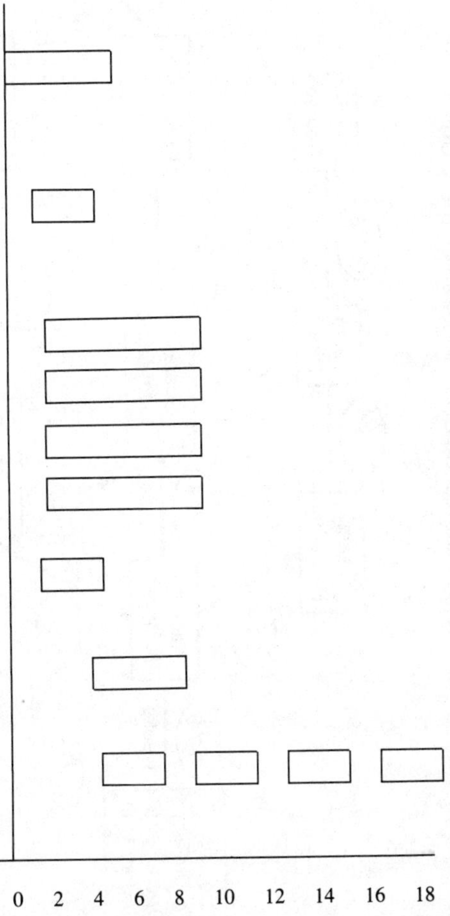

Months: 0   2   4   6   8   10   12   14   16   18

Figure 2-4 PERT Network for Renovation of Open-Heart Surgery Unit

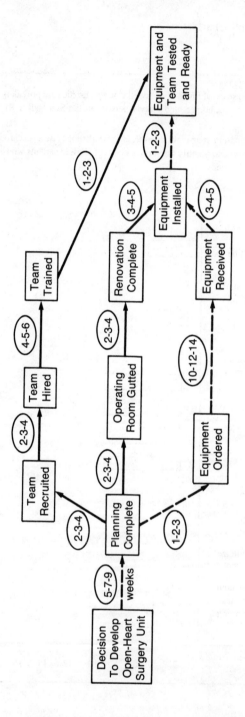

—— Critical Path

◯ weeks   Indicates in order of listing, estimates of most optimistic, most likely, and most pessimistic completion times

Source: From Beaufort Longest, Jr., *Management Practices for the Health Professional*, 3rd ed., 1984. Reprinted by permission of Reston Publishing Company, a Prentice-Hall Company, 11480 Sunset Hills Road, Reston, VA 22090.

several activities must be taking place simultaneously for PERT to be of any real value. This fact will become clear as we proceed.

To make the network understandable and usable, the time between the various events (activity time) must be computed. As anyone concerned with large-scale projects knows, it is not always possible to estimate accurately how long it will take to complete the various parts of the project. However, a method does exist whereby a fairly accurate estimated time between events can be determined. This approach involves estimating three different times for each activity:

1. *Optimistic Time*. This occasionally happens when everything goes right. The estimate is predicated on minimal and routine difficulties in the activity.
2. *Most Likely Time*. It represents the most accurate forecast based on normal developments. If only one estimate were given, this would be it.
3. *Pessimistic Time*. This is estimated on maximum potential difficulties. The assumption here is that whatever can go wrong will go wrong.

* * * * *

A formula based on the probability distribution of time involved in performing the activity is then used. The formula is:

$$\text{Activity Time} = \frac{O + 4M + P}{6}$$

Where O is optimistic time,
M is most likely time, and
P is pessimistic time.

Referring to Figure 2–4 , we can see that time estimates between the first two events have been made as follows: optimistic = 5 weeks, most likely = 7 weeks, and pessimistic = 9 weeks. The estimated activity time would then be:

$$t_e = \frac{5 + 4(7) + 9}{6} = 7 \text{ weeks}$$

Using the resulting value, we could be reasonably certain that the activity time between events 1 and 2 will be 7 weeks. The process of calculating activity time must be completed for all activities in the network.

The next step in applying the PERT approach is to determine the *Critical Path*. The Critical Path through the network is the path that takes the longest period of time to complete. In Figure [2–4] the Critical Path is shown by the dashed line. Inasmuch as the Critical Path takes the longest time and is the determinant of project completion, other events that do not lie along the Critical Path may be completed before the time they are actually needed. The time differential between scheduled completion of these noncritical events and the time when they are actually required to be completed is called the Slack Time. Where excessive Slack Time exists in the project or program, a reevaluation should take place. It should be determined which resources, and in what amounts, could be transferred to activities along the Critical Path. This may permit the Critical Path, and thus the completion time, to be shortened.

In our example, for instance, it would do no good to speed up recruitment, hiring, or training of the team or the renovation of the operating room *unless* we could reduce time on equipment delivery and installation. The entire process can be speeded up only through those activities since they form the Critical Path.[7]

When a disaster plan is in development, a number of events and activities will have to take place to ensure its completion. Among them are organizing a disaster planning committee, reviewing other plans, adopting a plan format, developing the disaster manual, reviewing first and second drafts of the plan and manual, conducting drills, and evaluating the outcome. PERT is an excellent tool for defining and managing this sequence. Figure 2–5 illustrates the use of PERT in doing so.

4. Responsibility Chart

A Responsibility Chart and a Resource Matrix are tools to use in detailing further the Scope-of-Work, Gantt, and PERT Charts. The Responsibility Chart provides a visual means for linking activity with personnel time and responsibility. Exhibits 2–8 and 2–9 illustrate use of the Resource Matrix to document personnel and other costs associated with the activities in Exhibits 2–6 and 2–7.

The Responsibility Chart specifies (1) who is responsible for each activity, (2) the roles (i.e., must be informed, primary responsibility, etc.), and (3) the

Figure 2–5 PERT Chart Illustration of Disaster Plan Development Sequence

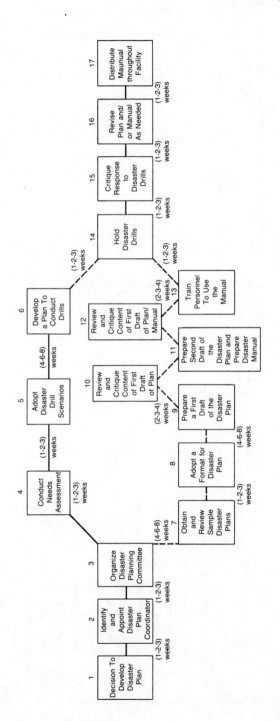

Exhibit 2–8 Example of Responsibility Chart

Objective: As a result of participation in an eight–hour training workshop series, 40 chronic care personnel will be able to identify the service needs of eligible disabled patients who are homebound during a disaster.

Personnel (job title or name) and Anticipated Time to Be Allocated

# Activities	Mary W., RN Disaster Coordinator		Alan A., MPH Hosp. Planner		Barbara J. SNF Administrator		Sandy R., PhD Health Educator	
	Role	Time	Role	Time	Role	Time	Role	Time
1.1 Assemble Advisory Committee	P	18 hrs.						
1.2 Prepare draft curriculum	C	2 hrs.			C	2 hrs.	P	6 hrs.
1.3 Advisory Committee								
a. Assess and critique curriculum	I	1 hr.	S	6 hrs.	S	6 hrs.	P	6 hrs.
b. Identify training workshop speakers			P	12 hrs.	C	2 hrs.	C	2 hrs.
c. Assess and critique evaluation instrument	S	2 hrs.	S	1 hr.	S	1 hr.	P	4 hrs.
d. Assist in publicizing training event	I	1 hr.	I	1 hr.	P	20 hrs.	I	1 hr.
1.4 Conduct telephone survey	P	30 hrs.					S	8 hrs.
1.5 Schedule and publicize training event	S	3 hrs.	S	3 hrs.	P	20 hrs.	S	3 hrs.
1.6 Conduct four two-hour training workshops in four locations throughout county	S	16 hrs.	C	2 hrs.	C	2 hrs.	P	16 hrs.

Role Responsibility:

I = Must be informed   C = Must be consulted
P = Primary responsibility   S = Provides support

Exhibit 2–9 Example of Resource Matrix

Objective: As a result of participation in an eight-hour workshop series, 40 chronic care personnel will be able to identify the service needs of eligible disabled patients who are homebound during a disaster.

Target Date:
1/1/87 Start-up
6/30/88 Complete

# Activities	Position	Role*	Time/ (hrs.)	Rate/hr.	Total Cost	Space	Rate	Equip.	Rate	Material	Rate	Activ. Total Cost	Target Date Completion
1.1 Assemble Advisory Committee	Disaster Coordinator	P	18	$21	$378	—	—	Tele-phone	$100	—	—	$478	1/1/87-3/31/87
	Hospital Planner	—	—	—									
	SNF Admin.	—	—	—									
	Health Educator	—	—	—									
1.2 Prepare Draft Curriculum	Disaster Coordinator	C	2	21	42	—	—	Word Pro-cessor	110	—	—	152	2/1/87-2/28/87
	Hospital Planner	—	—										
	SNF Admin.	C	2	22	44	—	—	Copy Machine	60	—	—	104	
	Health Educator	P	6	20	120	—	—	—	—	—	—	120	
1.3 Advisory Committee													
a. Assess and Critique Curriculum	Disaster Coordinator	I	1	21	21	Conf. Room Rental	150.	—	—	—	—	171	3/5/87-6/30/87
	Hospital Planner	S	6	24	144	—	—	—	—	Report	25	169	
	SNF Admin.	S	6	22	132	—	—	—	—	Report	25	157	
	Health Educator	P	6	20	180	—	—	—	—	Report	25	205	

Total cost: $1,556.

*I = Must be informed   C = Must be consulted
P = Primary responsibility   S = Provides support

expected amount of personnel time each activity will require. The Resource Matrix (Exhibit 2–9) provides a complete framework for costing out the completion of activities.

STEP 6: ACTION IMPLEMENTATION

This step in the problem-solving plan-development process instructs users on what to do. It is the action segment of the plan that specifies behavior expected, prescribing operating procedure for the entire organization as well as individual departments and units. (Chapter 4 details the outcomes of this step—the Disaster Manual.)

STEP 7: PLAN EVALUATION

The final step enables planners and users to examine whether or not the plan did what it was intended to do. Evaluation consists of comparing outcomes with the goal and objectives established at the beginning of the process. Standards that measure outcomes must be used. For example, the triage process can be evaluated by observing and timing performance during a drill. If an objective is to have triage fully operational within five minutes of notification, response times are a significant indicator of whether or not the objective was met.

There are two methods for selecting appropriate standards, each with its own advantages and disadvantages. One method is to involve potential users in deciding in advance on criteria or standards for success of the plan. Allowing them to set their own standard potentially motivates them to do a better job. The disadvantage is that their judgment will be biased and they gain little from failure. The alternative method is to consult experts, accrediting associations, and/or the literature for criteria. These standards can be said to be "objective." The disadvantage, however, is that standards applied elsewhere may not be appropriate for an individual facility.

SUMMARY

Planning is problem solving. The steps to planning discussed in this chapter are the same ones individuals take consciously and unconsciously to solve problems in their daily lives. Whether the problem is to buy new clothes for a summer vacation, ready a patient for satisfactory convalescence at home, successfully schedule and host a class reunion, or effectively manage the triage of mass casualties arriving after a train accident, the problem-solving process is the same.

The Planning Process   45

Problem solving involves seven steps: problem sensing, goal setting, needs assessment, objective setting, action plan detailing, action implementation, and plan evaluation. Each step requires information gathering, assessment, and decision. The steps build upon one another. Some plans involve elaborate needs assessment and action plan detailing, including charts and timetables. Others carry out the plan development process in a simpler manner.

The techniques described are by no means exhaustive. They are a sampling of the many practical tools available to disaster planners.

NOTES

1. Amitai Etzioni, *Modern Organizations* (Englewood Cliffs, NJ: Prentice-Hall, 1964), 5.

2. Olaf Helmer, "Analysis of the Future: The Delphi Method," in *Technological Forecasting for Industry and Government,* ed. James Bright (Englewood Cliffs, NJ: Prentice-Hall, 1968), 116–122.

3. Andrew Van de Ven and Andre Delbecq, "The Effectiveness of Delphi Interacting and Nominal Groups in Decision–Making Processes," *Academy Management Journal* 17, no. 4 (December 1974): 605–619.

4. Anthony Raia, *Managing by Objectives* (Glenview, IL: Scott, Foresman & Co., 1974), 24.

5. David Bergwell, Philip Reeves, and Nina Woodside, *Introduction to Health Planning* (Washington, DC: Information Resources Press, 1974), 80.

6. Ibid.

7. Beaufort Longest, Jr., *Management Practices for the Health Professional* (Reston, VA: Reston Publishing Co., 1980), 91–94.

REFERENCES

McConkey, Dale. *MBO for Nonprofit Organizations.* New York: American Management Association, 1975.

Maier, N.R.F. *Problem Solving and Creativity: In Individuals and Groups.* Monterey, CA: Brooks/Cole, 1970 .

Mitroff, I.I., Emshoff, J.R., and Kilmann, R.H. "Assumptional Analysis: A Methodology for Strategic Problem Solving." *Management Science* 25, no. 6 (June 1979): 583–593.

Nutt, P.C. "Hybrid Planning Methods," *Academy of Management Review* 7, no. 3 (July 1982): 443–454.

Shortell, S.M., and Richardson, W.C. *Health Program Evaluation.* St. Louis: The C.V. Mosby Company, 1980, 16–37.

Van Gigch, J.P. *Applied General Systems Theory.* New York: Harper & Row, 1974, 270–371.

Weinberg, G.M. *An Introduction to Systems Thinking.* New York: John Wiley & Sons, 1975.

Chapter 3

Beginning Work

The term "disaster" has as many definitions as people to define it. If health facilities are to develop a workable plan, a clear definition is necessary to focus planners on appropriate goals and objectives. Regardless of whether a disaster incident is man-made or natural, this definition should be event oriented and clinical. The American Red Cross identifies five categories of the most common disaster etiologies in order of occurrence: heat, cold, wind, fire, and earthquake.

All of these can cause psychological trauma and social dislocations as well as physical trauma. When "new age" disasters such as terrorism and hazardous chemical spills are considered as well, the etiology of disaster becomes complex indeed. Given the range of events, it is more useful to define disaster by its impact on the health care facility rather than by its cause:

> A disaster is any patient-generating incident which overloads existing personnel; or existing personnel, supplies, and equipment; or, which occurs in such magnitude that resources such as personnel, supplies, and equipment are not readily available for stabilization and treatment of casualties.[1]

PATIENT-GENERATING CRITERIA

It also is helpful to interpret a disaster in terms of the numbers of victims a facility can expect to receive rather than in terms of the types of injuries expected. The three patient-generating criteria developed by the Los Angeles County Medical Association provide such typology.[2] They divide into multiple patient, multiple casualty, and mass casualty incidents.

Multiple Patient Incident

This situation requires the response of two or more ambulances to the scene, but otherwise can be handled by the existing Emergency Medical Services System

(EMSS). Fewer than ten victims are generated and coordination of victim distribution by a county-coordinated communication center is not necessary, although it may occur. Time lags of 15 to 30 minutes between occurrence of the event and receipt of casualties at a health facility can be expected.

Multiple Casualty Incident

This event necessitates response of more than two ambulances and the coordination of casualty distribution by a coordinated communication center. The institution can expect a warning before the first victims arrive. The multiple casualty incident generates up to 50 victims, but the nature of the incident is limited in scope; the event seldom lasts more than a few hours. A time lag of 30 to 60 minutes between event occurrence and facility receipt of victims can be expected.

Mass Casualty Incident

While both a multiple casualty incident and a mass casualty incident require implementation of an organized field response that includes a disaster communication center, fire and police personnel, paramedics/emergency medical technicians (EMTs), and various community utility services, the true mass casualty incident overwhelms local resources. Mutual aid resources from outside the community are needed and, depending on the nature of the event, potentially state and federal assistance as well.

The mass casualty disaster can generate hundreds or thousands of victims, many of them seriously ill or injured, over hours, days, or even weeks. Although such an incident can involve a considerable time lag between occurrence and victim receipt, there may be little advance warning of arrival of the first casualty load. The waiting period (the time between the incident and receipt of first casualties) is fraught with psychological strain and the deleterious impact of rumors. Yet it also gives an opportunity for measured implementation of the facility disaster plan.

The problem of disaster response preparedness is complex, involving numerous factors. While natural and man-made disasters have dramatic consequences because they are a major cause of death, disability, and property loss, they are far from being exclusively a health problem. In fact, they are nonhealth problems with heavy health implications; hence the complex interaction among their various elements.[3]

Health facilities differ in the types of services available and their capabilities, resources, and location. Differing state and local requirements affect response. A workable disaster plan must consider the institution's unique characteristics. This is not to imply that there are no commonalities among facilities—there are many, of course. It is helpful to examine different plans, particularly those used by other facilities of comparable size and patient mix. This can save time, but it is not a panacea or short cut. Workable plans must be tailored to each facility.

Most disaster plans are prepared in two parts: one addresses external disasters, the other internal disasters. In all other ways (style, format, prescriptions for action) there invariably are differences. Some plans are elaborate hardbound documents, hundreds of pages in length; others are a compendium of statements, forms, and reports compiled in loose-leaf form and accompanied by only three or four pages of text. The suggestions proposed in this chapter were developed to complement the Joint Commission on Accreditation of Hospitals' (JCAH) disaster planning guidelines for hospitals. (See Appendix 4–A.)

THE DISASTER PLANNING COMMITTEE ROLE

While regulatory bodies do not require it, a disaster planning committee is essential to the development or revision of a disaster plan. Effective disaster planning cannot be accomplished by an individual. Few have the knowledge or the time to address all of the complexities. Unless representatives of key departments and outside organizations are involved in the planning, it will be difficult for them to endorse and comply with the plan wholeheartedly. While the panel must be of a reasonable and workable size, the following should be considered as its minimal membership.

Administration Representative

This individual must have sufficient authority to ensure compliance if any action is recommended. This representative should have sufficient planning experience and disaster training to be able to give expert assistance to the committee. When technical competence is coupled with authority, the plan has true potential for adoption and workability.

Medical Staff Representative

The institution's chief of staff or designee should be present at brainstorming and task review meetings of the committee. Although physician involvement is crucial in effective disaster response, too often facilities neglect to involve them in the nuts and bolts of developing the plan. Medical review, comment, and contribution all are vital to the clinical segments of a disaster plan. Physicians' ideas and needs must be incorporated. Many facilities rotate the medical staff representative role annually. This broadens medical involvement in plan development, plan review, and disaster training.

Nursing Department Representative

Nursing is central to an effective response. A representative of nursing administration should be an active member of the committee even if there are other nurses on the committee. Effective implementation and decision making during a disaster will have an impact on patient care areas and nursing functions throughout the facility, and this representative can be helpful in anticipating and solving problems related to these activities. During an actual disaster, the nursing department administrator will be critical to the coordination of patient care areas.

Emergency Department Representative

The emergency department is pivotal in disaster response. Decisions regarding which phase of implementation to initiate begin in the ED because it is the area that will have first contact with disaster field providers and with the disaster communication center(s) in the community. If the facility does not have a 24-hour ED (few SNFs have an ED and some hospitals do not staff their emergency receiving units around the clock), a representative of the department designated to receive disaster information from the community should be a member of the committee.

Engineering/Security/Maintenance Representatives

Critical elements of crowd control, media control, internal fire/flood hazards, facility stabilization, restriction of incoming persons, securing of doors and passageways, and the procurement and repair of equipment are elements that can be addressed only by involving those responsible for their management. Because these elements are integral to successful response to disaster, engineering, security, and maintenance representatives must be active participants in plan development, review, and practice.

If possible the disaster planning committee also should include representatives of these departments:

- social services
- housekeeping services
- psychological/chaplain services
- dietary
- central service
- personnel
- volunteer services
- community paramedic/fire/police services

These representatives may be permanent or ad hoc.

Members of the committee do not need advanced degrees or even prior training in planning. They do need a high level of interest in disaster planning and a motivation to attend meetings and complete work assignments. In addition, they need to be able to:

1. conceptualize ideas and futures
2. think logically and use the steps of problem solving appropriately
3. work well with others and have a participatory attitude
4. write reports and outline or abstract from reports
5. teach and motivate their colleagues.

Each member must be aware that the role of the committee is not merely review and approval; rather, it involves actual preparation (thinking, discussing, writing, critiquing) of the plan. Ad hoc members (technical consultants and community resource persons) must be told which meetings they are expected to attend and what they need to prepare in order to contribute to the discussions and deliberation. Specifying such expectations will better assure that the committee's work can be accomplished in a reasonable time. Ad hoc members also may be asked to forward work assignments to the committee for review and inclusion, whether or not they attend meetings.

Because of the committee's importance, representatives should have stature in the organization with formal influence over plan utilization. Otherwise, the plan is likely to be shelved as soon as it is completed. That means that for all practical purposes the facility will not have coordinated disaster drills or critiques. Without drills, it is doubtful whether the plan will be workable in the event of a disaster.

Disaster Planning Committee Chair

This position carries major importance because it is the one that influences, guides, coordinates, and implements the work of the committee. Some facilities limit the duties of the committee chairperson to the planning process and plan development, and assign others to tasks such as disaster coordination, disaster education, drill planning and implementation, and drill or event critique. Other institutions assign these responsibilities to a disaster coordinator, who not only chairs the committee but performs all of those tasks as well in a full time position.

The advantages of assigning one person to the role of disaster coordinator include the assurance of continuity and quality in disaster planning and preparedness. The following are recommended duties for the disaster coordinator:

1. reviewing existing plans (if any)
2. selecting disaster planning committee members

3. serving as disaster planning committee chair and coordinating meeting times and subcommittee work schedules
4. notifying committee members of meetings
5. editing and coordinating work projects for the committee
6. overseeing plan revision/development
7. overseeing compilation and distribution of the disaster manual
8. ensuring distribution of the revised/developed plan
9. conducting continuing education/training of all staff members (including attending medical staff)
10. providing orientation to the disaster plan and to the use of the disaster manual
11. managing responses to actual events: coordinating implementation of the plan, assessing needs, and progressively auditing plan utilization
12. planning, implementing, and conducting disaster drills
13. conducting informal and formal critiques of events and drills
14. identifying specialized experts from outside the facility to provide plan consultation where necessary
15. making monthly rounds to each department, evaluating disaster readiness, updating disaster manuals, identifying problems, and recommending corrective measures to the unit and to administration.

Costs may be higher and there is an increased risk of program fragmentation in facilities that divide these tasks among several persons. Given the many demands made upon managers in a health facility, disaster planning almost always receives lower priority attention. In the long run, designating one individual as a full time disaster coordinator is good planning and will save money.

COMMITTEE ACTIVITIES

To be effective, the disaster planning committee should meet on a regular basis. Depending on the workload, this requires twice-a-month meetings until the task of developing or revising a plan is completed. The committee then can meet bi-monthly to update the plan, revise the disaster manual, schedule and critique training, and so forth. Some facilities reassemble the committee only when a drill is to be held and for formal critiquing of drills and real events.

Because it is a formal committee, minutes must be maintained and available for review by administrative authorities, including regulatory bodies. The minutes should be distributed to members for review within a reasonable time after a meeting. Timely minutes are particularly important in assessing events and in reminding committee members of work assignments. The minutes should reflect any action to be taken, when, and by whom. Communication is essential if members are expected to complete assignments between meetings. An agenda distributed before the meeting date enables those responsible for a task to come prepared. At least once a year, both the minutes and agenda should reflect the review of current regulatory requirements and required action.

Specific activities of the disaster planning committee include:

1. disaster plan document review
2. disaster plan document revision
3. preparation of a statement of committee's goals/objectives for each year
4. review of new employee orientation to disaster readiness and response
5. drill scenario development
6. review of all written critiques
7. assistance in the development/review of the facility's and departmental disaster manuals
8. coordination of disaster plan activities with the management requirements of the facility's emergency department.

Criteria for evaluating committee operations are detailed in Exhibit 3–1.

HOSPITAL AND SNF GOALS

Because hospitals and SNFs are 24-hour, 365-days-a-year organizations, protection of inhouse patients as well as casualties received from a disaster is of paramount importance. As noted earlier, the three most critical goals of disaster operations in any health facility are:

1. rapid admission and treatment of casualties
2. initial and continuous medical care of casualties and seriously ill inpatients
3. protection of inpatients, with evacuation as required.

The disaster plan of the institution and of each of its units must be goal oriented and contain objectives designed to achieve goals within a practical framework. A statement of goals and the objectives for reaching each goal must be included in the facility Disaster Manual. Goals and objectives also are fundamental to every disaster drill. Unless goals and objectives are addressed consistently, it is easy to forget the purpose of disaster planning. Therefore, the disaster planning committee chair should restate the goals and objectives of each work session and the committee's role in achieving them.

While the committee must have the freedom to pace its work and to request assistance and other resources as necessary, without a successful startup even a well-intended committee may be doomed to failure. Exhibit 3–2 is an example of a startup checklist.

Exhibit 3–1 Disaster Planning Committee Operations Checklist

Committee Operation Criteria	Yes	No
1. Standing members include representatives from administration, nursing, safety/engineering, medical staff, emergency department, and support areas.		
2. Ad hoc members include representatives of entities outside the facility, from the fire department, police department, and other facilities.		
3. Committee members know their authority and responsibilities.		
4. Members have special training in disaster planning methods.		
5. Committee meetings are announced in advance, agendas are distributed, minutes are available.		
6. The committee has adequate clerical assistance.		
7. Meetings give ample opportunity for participation by everyone.		
8. New members are given adequate orientation training.		
9. Committee meetings are held in comfortable settings.		
10. The committee has a work schedule and timetable for action.		
11. Committee members are allowed time from their regular job assignments to do the work of the committee.		
12. The committee is the final arbiter for what ought to be included in/excluded from the plan document.		
13. The committee is active in disaster simulation training.		
14. The committee is active in the evaluation of disaster simulations.		
15. The committee reviews drill and event critiques within two weeks.		
16. The plan document is revised by the committee within three months of the critique.		

Developing a disaster plan is an evolving process. It brings together facility personnel, volunteers, representatives of public safety agencies, other health facilities, community groups of various kinds, and technical specialists. Because each institution is unique and because it serves a unique community, it is not possible to prescribe an activity sequence for developing or revising a disaster plan

Exhibit 3–2 Disaster Planning Committee Startup Checklist

Activities	*Date Completed*
1. Administration or Disaster Coordinator identifies standing and ad hoc members of Disaster Planning Committee.	
2. Administration selects temporary Disaster Planning Committee chairperson in advance of the first meeting.	
3. Temporary chair schedules the committee's first meeting.	
4. Temporary chair completes the agenda in advance of the first committee meeting.	
5. Temporary chair distributes the agenda in advance of the first meeting.	
6. Committee holds its first meeting and, at a minimum, completes the following tasks:	
a. defines the role of the committee	
b. introduces members to each other	
c. selects a permanent chairperson, who may be the Disaster Coordinator, and secretary (if a staff secretary is not available to record committee activity)	
d. chair and members establish goal(s) for the disaster plan	
e. chair and members establish objectives for each goal	
f. chair establishes subcommittees for each goal and assigns one or more committee members to each subcommittee	
g. chair establishes a timeline for the subcommittees to complete their work	
h. chair schedules the second meeting of the committee and prepares an agenda.	
7. Chair prepares detailed minutes and distributes them, along with the agenda, to committee members at least two days before the second meeting.	

that will work in every circumstance. Nevertheless there are milestones that should be considered. Figure 3–1 outlines a 150-day plan development and/or plan review process with 16 points that may be helpful.

The 150-day development process is generic. It will have to be modified to meet the unique needs of individual facilities; however, aspects of each of the 16 milestones will have to be addressed one way or another. The degree of completeness depends on a variety of factors, not the least of which is the assignment of a disaster coordinator to manage the entire process.

It is assumed that a plan can be completed within 90 days of startup, providing the subcommittees complete their work in gathering and collating data on their

Figure 3–1 150-Day Disaster Plan Development and Plan Review Process

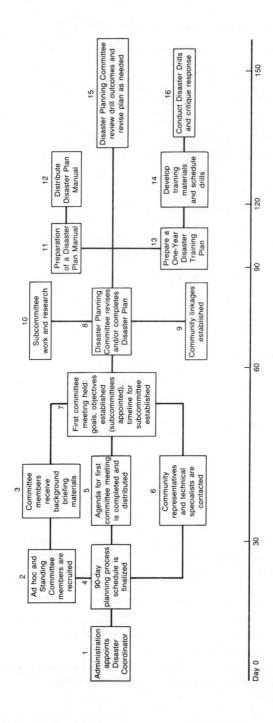

assigned tasks. Once milestone # 9 has been completed, the plan can become operational by preparing a disaster manual (# 11) and a disaster training plan (# 13). These two milestones are what make the plan workable. The manual prescribes specific roles for all facility units and designates procedures for mobilizing personnel (see Chapter 4). The training plan provides learning experiences for the prescriptions in the manual (see Chapter 5).

LINKING COMMUNITY RESOURCES IN PLANNING

It is important to include community agencies and other resources in the development of the facility plan document and in planning for and scheduling training activities. Fire and police agencies can assist in devising realistic drill scenarios that take into account the type of disaster that may reasonably be expected in various locales. Other agencies, such as the Red Cross, public utilities, National Guard, and airport authorities, are invaluable in developing both the plan and subsequent drill scenarios. Coordination with other agencies is vital in an actual event, and involving them in facility planning is the best way to assure this. In addition, every community has unused or underused resources that should be considered: ham radio operators, florists and their vehicles, mortuaries, etc. These may have much to offer. For example, when telephone lines are down, when the need for fast delivery of blood supplies arises, or when there is need for extra morgue space, several of these resources can prove invaluable.

Disaster planners must anticipate needs, then link them to resources. In the event of a mass casualty disaster, victims may have to be transported by city bus, taxi, moving van, etc. The facility and community must have established linkage with resources who, before any emergency, agree to respond to a call-up for assistance. Preplanning and agreements to coordinate are a must.

It also is important to link the institution to the area's Emergency Medical Services Systems agency or whatever unit of local government is responsible for community disaster response coordination. Virtually every county government in the nation has a community disaster plan. It is helpful to compare the facility's plan with the community's plan. The more collaborative they are with one another, the more likely that resources will be used effectively. Fire departments have their own plans that detail evacuation routes and other factors; law enforcement has plans for crowd and traffic control. These plans also should be considered in developing the facility's plan.

The institution's plan should specify the person(s) responsible for coordinating with public safety agencies as well as for contacting ambulance service companies to designate access routes to the facility when normal routes are closed. Care should be taken to include in the plan such items as entry and parking regulations, and procedures for handling the flow of rescue vehicles arriving and departing simultaneously.

Close collaboration with neighboring health facilities on evacuation procedures, receipt/transfer procedures, and mutual aid resources is imperative. So, too, is the simplification and standardization of paper work. The citywide or areawide use of identical forms and casualty tags can alleviate communication problems. The plan should specify the potential resources available from neighboring facilities and include methods for sharing such resources. To facilitate collaboration, a framework should be established for the health institutions to recover costs they incur in sharing supplies, equipment, and personnel when mutual aid is invoked.

Skilled nursing facilities may want to work with acute care hospitals in their area. Often overlooked, SNFs can be involved in receiving transferred patients from acute care hospitals if the latter have to empty beds to accommodate incoming casualties. Common transfer forms are beneficial in such circumstances.

Churches, National Guard armories, schools, and businesses can be integrated into the disaster plan. Prior agreements for mutual aid can anticipate a variety of needs: family relocation centers, additional food when the institution's own supplies are exhausted, and kitchen services in the event the facility's kitchen is damaged or otherwise nonfunctional. Pastoral assistance from local churches may be negotiated. These services are vital not only for casualties and survivors but also for staff members who are stressed by long work hours and who fear for the safety of family and friends.

If local schools, churches, larger stores, and industry do not have plans for action in the event of either internal or external disasters, health facilities should offer to help them develop such plans. Industry should be involved where appropriate, not only to consult in the development of plans for worker survival if no plan exists but also to establish procedures for utilization of resources. Hospitals and SNFs have needs similar to industry: plant safety, reduction of hazardous materials risks, and secure communications. Mutual needs are a real boost to collaboration.

Local medical societies should be consulted to determine the potential resources of physicians and specialist consultants. Some hospitals employ physicians. With few exceptions, every acute care hospital with 100 or more beds has at least one physician on duty inhouse 24 hours a day, particularly if they have an emergency department. Smaller hospitals and SNFs generally do not have physicians on duty.

In a disaster it is imperative that the facility coordinate physician resources. For that purpose, its own medical staff and the local medical society should be integrated into the planning process. Staff physicians must know what is expected of them. In a disaster that generates mass casualties, everyone who learns of it by whatever means will want to help. However, too much help, particularly if it is uncoordinated, actually is a hindrance. Therefore, health facilities require rapid but orderly response by all of their personnel, including physicians. Prior planning for this response will prevent problems.

The local medical society can be helpful in other ways, as well. Because its members use every facility in a community, it is in an excellent position to establish mass casualty physician response plans, multifacility blood bank and storage systems, and arrangements for back-up pharmaceutical supplies, to name but a few possibilities.

Finally, the plan should prescribe procedures for involving field triage personnel in the planning. For example, a consistent and uniform tagging system can be established to minimize confusion and triage errors when casualties arrive at receiving facilities. This may be a fairly simple system for small communities to agree upon. However, where communities are large and complicated by multiple jurisdictions, development of a tagging system coordinated between field providers and health facilities may be difficult. Uniform field triage tags are imperative, because lack of uniformity can be life threatening. Personnel can be familiarized with field triage materials and categories by involving as many as possible in mutual planning and drills.

Local law enforcement agencies should be consulted in developing a procedure for identifying health personnel who must travel to their workplaces. Without easily recognizable clothing, armbands, or IDs, these workers may find it impossible to cross police lines in the event of a major community disaster. California's Office of Emergency Services developed a system for emergency personnel to carry wallet cards containing their photo and identifying them as ''disaster service worker.'' This is intended to enable workers to cross police lines during a level III event (one that affects a county or region to the extent that state resources are mobilized).

SUMMARY

The key to effective disaster planning is in organizing the planning function. A disaster planning committee composed of representatives of departments from throughout the institution is fundamental to that planning effort. The committee should be augmented on an ad hoc basis by specialists from the facility's service community: police, fire, Red Cross, etc. The committee's role is to develop the facility plan, develop a disaster manual based upon the plan, oversee disaster preparedness training, and conduct formal critiques of the responses in all training or actual disaster events.

A full-time disaster coordinator is recommended. Among other attributes, the individual's knowledge of planning methods and of disaster issues and problems, as well as strong leadership skills, are important. The disaster coordinator provides program continuity and technical expertise. If that role is divided among several persons, it tends to become diluted and planning suffers accordingly.

A generic 150-day planning and training process can assist planners in developing disaster preparedness programs. While many components may not be appropriate for every facility, aspects of each of them will be. The disaster planning committee should involve community resources to enrich the planning process and to establish firm linkages that can be depended upon during an actual disaster.

NOTES

1. Joan Kelley Simoneau, "Disaster Management," in *Emergency Nursing: Principles and Practices*, 2d. ed., ed. Susan A. Sheehy and Janet M. Barber (St. Louis: The C.V. Mosby Company, 1985).

2. Los Angeles County Medical Association Bulletin, *Disasters—Procedural Guideline for Triage Medical Officer* (December 1977).

3. California Governor's Earthquake Task Force, "Sociological Aspects of Disasters" (Sacramento, CA, 1982). Unpublished report.

REFERENCES

American Hospital Association. *Principles of Disaster Preparedness for Hospitals*. Chicago: American Hospital Association, 1956.

———. *Readings in Disaster Planning for Hospitals*. Chicago: American Hospital Association, 1966.

Cohen, Eddi. *Disasters! An Emergency Care Workbook*. San Diego: Instructional Development and Educational Aids, Inc., 1982.

Cohen, Raquel. *Handbook for Mental Health Care of Disaster Victims*. Baltimore: Johns Hopkins University Press, 1980.

Foster, Harold. *Disaster Planning: The Preservation of Life and Property*. New York: Springer Publishing, 1981.

Healy, Richard. *Emergency and Disaster Planning*. New York: John Wiley and Sons, 1969.

Jenkins, Astor and vern de Leuv, John, eds. *Emergency Department Organization and Management*. St. Louis: The C.V. Mosby Company, 1978.

Noble, J.H., Wechsler, H., La Montagne, M., and Noble, M. *Emergency Medical Services: Behavioral and Planning Perspectives*. New York: Behavioral Publications, 1973.

Savage, Peter. *Disasters: Hospital Planning*. Oxford: Pergamon Press, 1979.

Thygerson, Alton. *Disaster Survival Handbook*. Salt Lake City: Brigham Young University Press, 1979.

Chapter 4

The Disaster Manual

Chapter 3 described how planners can use a seven-step process to develop and implement a plan. That process is generic to planning of any kind, including disaster planning.

As described earlier, disaster plans differ from other plans in one vital way: they are written to prepare the facility to respond to the demands of an uncontrollable event and not to control events as do other types of plans.

> Most hospitals have disaster plans that provide for people *coming* to the hospital during a crisis when the hospital is not physically involved . . . . But what does the hospital do when it is as hard hit as the community?[1]

This question highlights the challenge facing health facilities. They must prepare for disasters affecting either the institution itself, its service community, or both.

Some plans use considerable narrative; others, charts to depict expected relationships for personnel and programs; still others, merely outlines of expected events and responsibilities. There are no standards other than that each plan must be usable by the facility involved. In a disaster, logic and certainty are at a premium and can be lifesaving. A realistic plan and a readable manual can make the difference.

Most disaster plans are prepared in two parts, one concerned with external and the other with internal events. The former focuses on receipt of casualties and their distribution in the facility, the latter on inhouse patients and staff as well as damage to the facility. Both parts emphasize response procedures and assignments for personnel. The Joint Committee on Accreditation of Hospitals (JCAH) is prescriptive about what each part ought to contain.[2] Its requirements are reprinted in Appendix 4–A at the end of this chapter.

Many SNFs follow JCAH guidelines voluntarily, but they also must comply with state and local regulations, which vary considerably. The *Administrative Code of the State of California* offers comprehensive disaster plan standards for SNFs (Appendix 4-B).

Many facilities distinguish between internal and external plans. However, there is a danger in doing so, particularly if in training for one type of event, the other is overlooked as occurred in the case of one facility. Struck by a sizable earthquake, an acute care community hospital in one California city was both the rescuer and victim. Dozens of persons were injured when the ceiling in a discount store collapsed on preholiday shoppers. The quake also interrupted power and telephone service to the hospital, and for an unrelated reason the facility's own electrical generator was inoperable at the time. When casualties started arriving—many walked in or drove in themselves—hospital personnel were busy trying to evacuate inhouse patients. The resultant confusion at the 95-bed facility and the bottleneck it created for the handful of ambulances available was considerable. In a postdisaster critique it was determined that persons involved had been working at cross-purposes with one another. For instance, the nursing director and emergency physician simultaneously, but independently, authorized startups for the internal and external plans. It took nearly 30 minutes to unsnarl patient reception and evacuation traffic. The problem was exacerbated by inoperable elevators and a lack of telephones for interdepartment communication.

Disaster planning should result in two outcomes: (1) It should prepare the facility to respond effectively to a disaster event, and (2) it should result in the production of a readable, easily understood *Disaster Manual*.

The *Disaster Manual*, with minor modifications, is a compilation of the fifth, sixth, and seventh steps of the problem-solving process (Figure 4–1). When the plan is updated subsequently (usually every year) the problem-solving process should be used again and the manual modified accordingly.

Figure 4–1 Relationship of Problem-Solving Process to Disaster Manual

Problem-Solving Planning Process

Step 1 Problem Sensing

Step 2 Goal Setting

Step 3 Needs Assessment

Step 4 Objective Setting

Step 5 Action Plan Detailing

Step 6 Action Implementation   **Disaster Manual**

Step 7 Plan Evaluation

MODEL DISASTER MANUAL

Disaster manuals are assembled in a variety of ways; however, most have 14 major sections. Those sections are treated in this chapter as a model. A table of contents for the manual is presented in Exhibit 4–1. Each of its 14 sections is analyzed below.

Section I Plan Implementation

The plan implementation section of the manual should contain seven subsections:

1. Table of Contents
2. Letter of Authorization
3. Community/Regional/Facility Casualty Philosophy Statement
4. Collaborating Agencies/Facilities Statement
5. Goal/Objectives Statement
6. Definition of Terms/Decision Criteria
7. Notification Procedure.

The plan implementation section prescribes general response procedures to be followed once word is received of a disaster event (internal or external).

One fundamental decision to be made in any disaster is when and how to initiate facility response. The basic element in this decision is how valid the disaster report is. The plan implementation section must define the levels and/or categories of disaster and the manner in which the person discovering it or being notified of it is to activate the facility.

Each subsection of the Plan Implementation section is discussed next.

1. Table of Contents

See Exhibit 4–1 for an example of a model *Disaster Manual* table of contents.

2. Letter of Authorization

This document, a signed and dated memo or letter, formally authorizes the actions prescribed in the manual. It sometimes includes a statement of philosophy, as well. (Exhibit 4–2 is an example.) The authorization for use should be among the first materials in the manual.

3. Community/Regional/Facility Casualty Philosophy Statement

This defines how the facility will interrelate with community and regional disaster operations and its philosophy on casualty disbursement and receipt. The

Exhibit 4–1 Table of Contents for a Model Disaster Manual

I. Plan Implementation

   1. Table of Contents
   2. Letter of Authorization
   3. Community/Regional/Facility Casualty Philosophy Statement
   4. Collaborating Agencies/Facilities Statement
   5. Goal/Objectives Statement
   6. Definition of Terms/Decision Criteria
   7. Notification Procedure

II. Personnel Notification

   1. Chain of Command
   2. Notification
   3. Callback Procedure

III. Command Post

   1. Opening the Command Post
   2. Staffing and Equipment

IV. Personnel Pool

   1. Function
   2. Staffing and Equipment
   3. Procedures

V. Communications

   1. Function
   2. Staffing and Equipment
   3. Procedures

VI. Paper Work and Forms

VII. Triage Area

   1. Function
   2. Staffing and Equipment
   3. Procedures

VIII. Major Treatment Area

   1. Function
   2. Staffing and Equipment
   3. Procedures

IX. Delayed Care Area

   1. Function
   2. Staffing and Equipment
   3. Procedures

X. Departmental Responsibilities

   Accounting/Data Processing
   Admitting (Inpatient and Outpatient)

Exhibit 4–1 continued

Administration
Business Office
Central Service
Clergy
Dietary/Food Services
Disaster Coordination
Emergency Department
Housekeeping
Infection Control
Laboratory
Laundry
Materials Management
Medical Records
Medical Staff
Mental Health
Morgue
Nuclear Medicine
Nursing Service
Nursing Units
Outpatient Services
Pathology
Personnel
Pharmacy
Physical Therapy
Plant Operations/Engineering
Public Relations
Purchasing
Radiology
Respiratory Therapy
Security
Social Services
Surgery/Recovery
Switchboard
Volunteer Services

XI. Internal Disaster

1. Fire Procedures
2. Patient Evacuation Procedures
3. Physical Plant Damage Control
    Power Supply
    Gas Supply
    Water Supply

XII. Community Interface

1. Media Relations Center/Public Information Center
2. Public Safety
3. Ambulance
4. Red Cross and Other Agencies

Exhibit 4–1 continued

XIII. Special Incidents

    Bomb Threat
    Severe Weather
    Earthquake
    Terrorism
    Hazardous Chemical
    Radiation
    Civil Disorder

XIV. Attachments

    1. Disaster Training Plan
    2. Cost-Recovery Procedures
    3. Long-Term Disaster Response
    4. Managing the Stress of Disaster
    5. Evacuation Maps/Instructions
    6. Location of Shut-Off Valves

statement should identify briefly the general procedure for field disbursement of casualties as conducted by organized emergency response teams. A general review of where the community disaster communications center will be and how it will assist in organized triage should be included. If the community's institutions

Exhibit 4–2 Sample Letter of Authorization

August 1, 19___

To: All Hospital Personnel
From: Chief Executive Officer
Subject: HOSPITAL DISASTER PLAN
         AUTHORIZATION POLICY

Policy Number: 10
Effective Dates: 8/___ - 7/___

A disaster can occur without warning. Flexible response is imperative. We must be prepared to provide any and all of the assistance that we can and to handle a large influx of victims regardless of the time, size, character, or duration of the emergency.

This plan was developed to guide our response. All personnel must be familiar with the plan as described in this manual, and with their specific responsibilities.

Each department manager is responsible for ensuring the adequate preparation of personnel before a disaster. Departmental plans support the overall Hospital Disaster Plan and must be followed.

are divided into receipt groups, this statement should define how these groups are identified and in what way they will be utilized.

4. Collaborating Agencies/Facilities Statement

The statement on casualty disbursement and receipt should be followed by a listing of state/regional/community agencies with which the institution may relate. A brief description of their function is appropriate. Possible collaborating agencies/facilities include:

County Disaster Communication Center
Emergency Agencies
  Police
  Fire
  Civil Defense
  Red Cross
  State Emergency Medical Authority
  Federal Emergency Management Agency
Transportation
  Ambulance Services
  Hospital Vans
  Florist Trucks
Facilities Receiving Evacuated Patients
  Acute Care Hospitals
  Skilled Nursing Facilities

This section statement should not include contact person names or telephone numbers; instead, it should identify the location where the list of names and current telephone numbers can be found.

5. Goal/Objectives Statement

This is a restatement of the goal and objectives used in developing the disaster plan. The objectives are targets to be achieved in training and in actual response (Exhibit 4-3).

6. Definition of Terms/Decision Criteria

Materials and instructions for this subsection should define when and under what circumstances a disaster situation should be declared. Some commonly used code definitions and action steps are itemized in Exhibit 4-4.

Exhibit 4–3 Sample Goal and Objectives Statement

Goal:
> The goal of X Hospital's 1989-91 Disaster Plan is to enable the hospital to respond rapidly to mass casualties from throughout the city.

Objectives:
1. The hospital will be ready to receive both immediate and delayed casualties from a disaster site within 15 minutes of the initial alert.

2. The hospital will continue to provide nursing and medical care to inpatients during a disaster situation for at least two weeks after notification.

3. The hospital will be able to evacuate at least 50 percent of existing inpatients smoothly and safely, within one hour of notice, to appropriate facilities.

---

7. Notification Procedure

This formal policy statement gives the facility's rationale for service and procedures for announcing the disaster. It can be prepared as a memo, diagram with accompanying narrative, or in some similar format. It should designate those responsible for the announcement, the circumstances for making it, and how it can be cancelled.

This component of the plan must detail concisely the manner in which the person discovering or being notified of the event will activate the institution. Figure 4–2 outlines a notification sequence followed in an acute care hospital.

The response capability of a facility during a disaster depends on its capacity. If an institution has an emergency department (ED), it probably is able to respond routinely to "minidisasters" that might swamp a facility with no ED or with one that is quite small. Minidisasters are not unusual, but even a large ED may be capable of only a marginal response until off-duty personnel arrive to assist if it is near capacity when the disaster occurs.

If the facility has an ED, it is wise to consider a phased, or stepwise, implementation of disaster response to meet the demands both of multiple victim and of multiple casualty incidents. In the event the patient load overtaxes staff for any reason—disaster or nondisaster (which may include a lack of beds in the hospital, resulting in increasing numbers of patients waiting and being monitored in the ED until beds are ready)—certain elements of the disaster plan may be activated. In many cases, merely calling back one or two department staff members may resolve the crisis. The term "phasing" is sometimes used to describe such implementation. Phasing involves a minimum staff callback at certain numbers of arriving or expected patients, opening of the Triage Area at certain numbers, opening of the department Command Post at certain numbers, and so forth.

This stepwise implementation for disaster operations requires the development of:

1. Steps for phasing in the facility/department plan based on preestablished numbers and/or acuity.
2. Clear designation of who will be expected to make the decision on the initial implementation level and increasing the level; and how, and to whom, that decision will be communicated.
3. Detailed instructions for the ways in which various departments must alter their routine work during the phasing.

An example of a phasing plan in a hospital manual follows:

Phase	No. of Casualties	Units To Activate Initially
Phase 1	1-10	ED, Lab, X-ray
Phase 2	10-20	All of the above plus Triage Area, Delayed Care Area, ED Command Post, Hospital Command Post
Phase 3	20-50	All of the above plus Surgery, Critical Care Units, morgue, personnel pool
Phase 4	50 +	Full plan implementation, including potential inhouse patient transfer.

Individual department manuals (see Department Responsibilities section below) should complement the overall facility manual and be integrative for stepwise implementation to be successful. Some facilities announce the phasing sequence on the public address system to alert departments of the disaster mode and trigger specific predetermined departmental reaction.

Section II Personnel Notification

This section details specific procedures. It consists of three subsections:

1. Chain of Command
2. Notification
3. Callback Procedure.

1. Chain of Command

Generally, an organization chart is used in the manual to identify key administrative and clinical personnel and their authority relationships. Because personnel turnover can be frequent, titles rather than individuals should be listed. The

Exhibit 4–4 Example of Code Definitions and Action Steps

Action Code and Type of Event	Definitions	Action Steps
CODE: WHITE Type: Tornado	Condition Standby (Impending in the county)	1. Close drapes 2. Open windows approximately 12 inches 3. Move patients and visitors away from windows 4. Keep patient doors OPEN
	Condition Stat (Hospital or immediate area)	1. IMPLEMENT FULL DISASTER PLAN 2. Move ambulatory patients to shower stalls with pillow over head 3. Protect head and chest of nonambulatory patients with pillows and move them into hall
	Condition All Clear	1. No danger—resume normal activity
CODE: GREEN Type: Mass Casualties	Condition Standby (Casualties under rescue)	1. Notify Administrator or Administrator on call 2. Begin calling from priority list
	Condition Stat (Casualties here or en route)	1. IMPLEMENT FULL DISASTER PLAN 2. All of above plus notify the chiefs of Surgery and Medicine
	Condition All Clear	1. No danger—resume normal activity

CODE: BLACK
Type: Bomb

Condition Standby
(Threat or suspected)

1. Give suspected location
2. Evacuate immediate area
3. Notify police, hospital Administrator, and Clinical Coordinator

Condition Stat
(Actual bomb)

1. IMPLEMENT FULL INTERNAL DISASTER PLAN
2. Evacuate under the direction of Administration

Condition All Clear

1. No danger—resume normal activity

CODE: RED
Type: Fire

Condition Standby
(Drill or suspected)

1. Give location
2. Close all doors
3. Respond to area with fire extinguishers

Condition Stat
(Actual hospital fire)

1. IMPLEMENT FULL INTERNAL DISASTER PLAN
2. Pull lever to notify Fire Department
3. Confine fire
4. Evacuate from areas near fire
5. Administration directs FULL evacuation

Condition All Clear

1. No danger—resume normal activity

Figure 4–2 Sample Disaster Notification Sequence

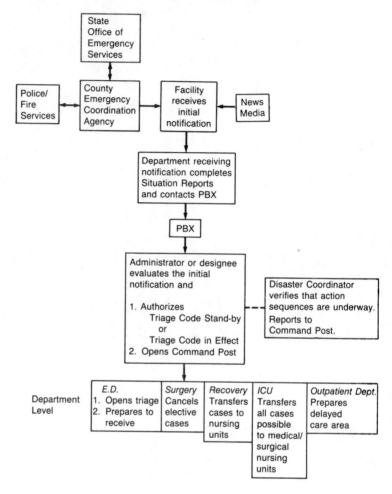

purpose of the chart is to familiarize personnel with the administrative hierarchy and linkages responsible for action.

2. Notification

This subsection includes such elements as:

• levels, or stages, of implementation, depending on the extent of the emergency

- an explicit explanation of public address system codes
- the procedure for announcing a disaster, including:
  a. who will announce
  b. under what circumstances
  c. how it will be announced
  d. who will cancel the announcement
  e. under what circumstances the announcement will be cancelled
  f. who will terminate disaster response activities.

Exhibit 4–5 is an example of a decision chart detailing expected responses. When the situation is external to the institution, the decision to define an event as a real or potential disaster depends upon a number of variables:

- notifier of the facility (public safety agency? Disaster Communication Center? citizen?)
- ability to verify the disaster
- type of disaster and numbers of casualties the facility can anticipate receiving
- current facility census
- current Emergency Department census
- time of day, day of week (personnel available)
- physical integrity of the facility (damage).

The person receiving initial notification must have a procedure to follow for verification, unless the incident is being communicated over an interhospital radio network or computer system (Exhibit 4–6). That person also must have a procedure for notifying the ranking administrator on duty so decisions can be made regarding the level to activate the facility. In the event the ED will be receiving only a small number of casualties, the institution may decide to alert Surgery to clear only one operating suite, for example, or Lab and X-ray to call in one or two staff persons to assist with victim evaluation.

If the facility has an ED, information on an external disaster has a tendency to filter into that department before administration or even the switchboard operator can learn of it. The ED unit manual must define how the on-duty physician and nurse determine to what degree to mobilize and when to involve the administrator or nursing supervisor. In many cases, stepwise implementation of the ED plan should precede implementation of the inhouse plan.

Even so, notification of a ranking administrative person should never be neglected. If such notification is not made, the situation may escalate and overwhelm the ED and vital inhouse backup services and resources will not be ready when needed. It is critical that the ED physician and RN on duty know how to determine signs of staff overload before the problem gets out of hand and that they

Exhibit 4–5 Example of Decision Criteria—Outcomes Chart

Type	Code	Code Activated by	Notification	Response
External				
Any problem external to the facility resulting in the arrival of numbers of ill or injured persons	Green (minor) 0-10 casualties	On-duty Administrator in concert with ED physician and RN on duty	Nursing Office, Surgery, ICU, Lab, X-ray	ED Triage and Major Treatment areas readied
	Yellow (intermediate) 10-20 casualties	On-duty Administrator	Same as above and CEO, chief of staff	ED Triage Area, ED Command Post, and Major and Minor Treatment areas open
	White (major) 20+ casualties and/or major external disaster of continuous nature	On-duty Administrator	Same as above, plus all department personnel	All departments; evaluate inhouse patients for discharge and/or evacuation, activate only upon direct order by hospital Command Post

Internal

Any problem that puts patients at risk and disrupts or has the potential for disrupting routine:	Green (minor)	On-duty Administrator	Chief of staff, CEO, ED physician on duty, Nursing Office	Rescue and treatment in facility
fire	Yellow (intermediate)	On-duty Administrator	As above plus medical and clinical staff, nearby health facilities, public safety agencies, county disaster coordination center	Rescue, treatment, and/or evacuation
smoke				
explosion				
hazardous chemical				
structure damage				
power failure	White (major)	On-duty Administrator	As above plus Red Cross, community disaster agency	Evacuation
failure of communication equipment				
bomb threat	Red (fire)			
hostage situation				

Exhibit 4–6 Disaster Notification Form

Initial form for description of event when first notification is received. TRY TO OBTAIN ALL PERTINENT INFORMATION SO THAT APPROPRIATE RESPONSE CAN BE DETERMINED PROPERLY.

Date _____ Time _____ A.M./P.M.
Person Taking Report: _____ Position: _____
Area Where Notification Is Received: _____

    Name of Person Contacting: _____
    Agency: _____
    Call Originating From: _____ Phone # _____
    Verified: Yes/No   Comment _____

Nature of Event: (circle)

    Wind   Fire   Rain   Flood   Explosion   Bomb Threat
    Chemical (type) _____ Heat   Cold
    Vehicular (type) _____ Aircraft (type) _____
    Other: _____

Location: _____

Estimated Number of Casualties: (circle)
    1-6   6-10   10-20   20-30   30-40   40-50   50-60   60-70
    70-100   more than 100   more than 200
    Comment _____

Types of Injuries Prevailing: _____
_____

Numbers This Facility Should Expect:
    _____ Immediate _____ Delayed
    Comment: _____

Distribution Flow of Casualties Initially: _____
_____
_____

Additional Information:

White: Command Post/Administration. Pink: Area receiving notification.

be able to use specified criteria to determine the degree to which the facility must mobilize. Such criteria must be developed before an event and be included in the manual, including such elements as:

- Is the event multiple patient, multiple casualty, or mass casualty?
- Is the number of casualties known (to a reasonable degree)?
- Is the magnitude of the event likely to generate victims over an extended period or will receipt of casualties be limited to a manageable number over a short time?
- What type of injuries are involved?
- Can the ED control the number of casualties (both critical and noncritical) that the institution will receive either by direct communication with field triage or through a county disaster communication center?
- How many staff members and patients are present in the ED now?
- Does the time of day/day of week support obtaining staff quickly?
- How many beds are:
  —immediately available in the ED?
  —potentially available within 15 minutes?
  —potentially available within 30 minutes?
- How is the general equipment/supply status in the ED right now?

3. Callback Procedure

The procedure in the manual defines the method of callback; it may consist of a narrative instruction sheet, a callback roster, or both. In some facilities the PBX operator makes the calls, while in others they are the responsibility of the department heads or their designee(s).

Once notified, the Administrator's first actions should be to confirm the event, then to notify the Disaster Coordinator and department heads. Notification lists in disaster manuals range from a pyramid list with one caller making all calls (e.g., PBX operator) to a fanout calling list with each individual called in turn calling a few other specified persons.

The callback procedure in the manual indicates the manner in which the calling should be performed. A sample list as well as sample blank callback forms should be included in this subsection. The actual callback work sheet should be separated from the manual and kept with disaster supplies so that personnel can locate them and begin working without having to refer to the manual (Exhibit 4–7). It also is helpful to have the callback lists, which can be updated and revised easily, include the names and current telephone numbers; sample lists in the manual indicate titles or fictitious personnel only. In this way the procedure will not have to be revised in the manual every time there is a change in personnel.

Exhibit 4-7 Sample Staff Call Roster for Disaster

Name	Telephone No.	Time called	Response WBI*	Response No	Response No Ans.	ETA	Time Arrived	Comments
Sample, Joe	323–1111	10:40	X			5 min.	10:53	
Jones, John	874–8833	10:42		X				Road inaccessible; he will come in when situation changes.
Smith, Jane	342–8351	10:45		X				Mother states she is out of town.
Lindsey, Roberta	395–6458	10:46	X			15 min.	11:00	

*WBI = Will Be In

Source: Reprinted from "Disaster Management" by J.K. Simoneau in Emergency Nursing: Principles and Practice, 2nd ed. S.A. Sheehy and J.M. Barber (Eds.), with permission of the C.V. Mosby Company. St. Louis, © 1985.

While notification work sheets for supervisory personnel can be compiled in any format, including alphabetical, the main consideration should be that the list is easily understood and usable.

It is useful to prepare a callback roster with geographic areas shaded to indicate residential distance from the facility in 5-mile, 10-mile, and 15-mile radius increments. Those living farthest away would be contacted last because their travel time alone precludes their being of any immediate support. In addition, a disaster affecting an entire community may well result in closed roads. The closest staff members thus are more likely to be able to return to the facility while those farther away may not. It is helpful to divide the callback roster by shifts and to begin calling personnel already scheduled to return at the next change of shift because they are more likely to be available. There must be some mechanism for continuity of calling or transfer of responsibility for calling so that everyone looking at the form is aware immediately of who has been called, when, and the result (i.e., returning to work, not at home at time of call, etc.).

Many facilities assign callback responsibilities to either the Command Post or the switchboard operator. Whoever is assigned should have updated callback work sheets.

Callback rosters should be prepared in duplicate so that, once calls have been completed, a copy can be forwarded to the Command Post for tracking of returning personnel. Callback sheets should be updated quarterly to verify telephone numbers—more frequently if the rosters are linked to work schedules.

Equally important is the need for a procedure for off-duty personnel to initiate as soon as they become aware that a disaster affecting the facility has occurred. For example, this procedure may include a directive asking that they keep their home phone line unused when they learn of a disaster. The directive may indicate how, if at all, television and radio stations will be used to notify employees to return, and what stations to tune in.

Notification of physician staff is a critical element that must be incorporated into the manual, regardless of whether physicians are employed by the institution or serve as private attending staff. Developing a usable call list of physicians will depend upon how many of them are responsible to other facility or agency disaster responses and what types of doctors will be needed. Identifying medical specialty needs is very important—the physician(s) who will serve as ED Triage Officer(s) are the obvious example, but others, such as general surgeons, are equally important. Their assignments should be predefined.

Ensuring that physicians who respond are familiar with the manual and the facility is a must. If physicians respond in large numbers to an affected facility during a disaster, serious problems can result: they may be challenged by security personnel who, unless otherwise authorized, will deny them access. They may not know where to go in the hospital, including where the MD pool is located. Without an ID and in the tumult of a disaster, walk-in physicians may disrupt rather than help, and may in fact be turned away. The manual (and the disaster planners) thus must address these questions:

- Who will provide medical direction to physician responders in a disaster?
- What systems need to be developed to ensure physician callbacks, assignments based on area of expertise, authentication and identification of outside medical personnel, granting of temporary privileges, identification of alternate physicians to established department medical directors, and procedures for continuation of medical care to inpatients.
- How will physicians be made aware of all policies/procedures in the *Disaster Manual* that affect medical care and operations? What system will ensure continuing training on revisions? How will new medical staff members receive exposure to the plan?
- Who will be responsible for updating the Medical Staff Disaster Roster and how often?

Exhibit 4–8 is a sample of a physician callback procedure to be included in the manual.

Section III Command Post

This section of the manual details:

1. How the Command Post is to operate
2. How it should be staffed and equipped.

The Command Post is the institution's nerve center in a disaster. Therefore, it should be located in an easy-to-find, easily accessible location. The equipment—desks, wall charts, direct-line telephones, files—should be dedicated solely to its use. Anticipating physical damage to the facility, a secondary (backup) Command Post location should be identified. (The fire department may require that the Command Post be on the first floor of the facility.)

In preparing procedures for the Command Post section, a number of questions should be considered:

- Is its location central and is an alternate location designated in the event the primary area is damaged, unsafe, or inaccessible?
- Have equipment/supply lists been developed that are reasonable, functional, and obtainable in a disaster? Is auxiliary emergency power available? Are Command Post telephone lines direct linkages and separate from outside telephone lines (which may be inoperable)?

Exhibit 4–8 Sample Physician Callback Procedure

POLICY

It is the responsibility of the hospital to provide physicians for the treatment of casualties generated from a disaster event and received by our hospital.

PROCEDURE

1. Once Code Triage has been initiated, one staff member designated by the charge nurse of the Emergency Department (ED) will notify the ED Medical Director or designee to authorize ED physician callback.

2. Once Code Triage is in effect, the ED physician on duty will act as the physician in charge until the ED Medical Director or designee arrives.

3. The ED physician in charge will determine the number of ED and attending staff physicians to be called back, depending on the number and type of casualties anticipated.

4. The ED physician in charge will notify Medical Staff Office if dispatching available senior residents to the ED is warranted.

5. The ED clerk will initiate on-call specialty physician contacts upon the order of the ED physician in charge.

6. Physicians contacted directly by the ED will report to the ED.

7. If and when the hospital command post opens, contact work sheets will be sent there for continuation of contact and follow-up.

8. Physicians contacted by the Hospital Command Post and/or who hear of a disaster through the media will report to Medical Personnel Pool to await assignment.

- Have alternative means of communication been defined in the event all telephone lines are nonfunctional?
- Are there clearly defined procedures and criteria for activating the Command Post, including who will activate it and who will be responsible for its operations? Have appropriate personnel been assigned to the Command Post? At a minimum, these should include the CEO or Administrator, the Director of Nursing or Nursing Administrator, the Chief of the Medical Staff, and the designated facility Disaster Coordinator. If a Disaster Medical Officer position is established, this person also should be assigned to the Command Post.
- Has a Function and Staffing profile been included in the manual (see Exhibit 4–9) and is it available as a work sheet?
- What will be done to ensure the safety and security of the area? How will authorized personnel be identified prior to entry?

Exhibit 4–9 Example of Command Post Activation Procedure

COMMAND POST

Location: Conference Room 3, adjacent to Administrator's office

Personnel Assigned: Chief Executive Officer
Associate Administrator, Patient Care Services
Assistant Administrator, Allied Health Services
Chief, Medical Staff
Disaster Coordinator
Director of Security
Secretary
Messenger

Statement of Responsibilities
The Command Post will:

1. provide incident-related information to news media
2. monitor external emergency radio communication
3. coordinate facility response with other hospitals and agencies
4. coordinate all intrahospital activities
5. maintain call rosters for personnel and track staff on duty
6. receive and maintain data regarding response operations both inside and outside the facility
7. authorize discharge/transfer of house patients
8. update and revise Disaster Patient Master List and provide copies to Admitting, PBX, Public Relations.

- Have procedures been outlined for reports and other documents to be delivered to the Command Post and compiled and updated to provide management with an accurate assessment of the facility's status? (Some facilities assign personnel as Command Post messengers to assure document delivery.)
- Have procedures been established for securing the facility's computer, data base, and files? A power failure can knock out large and small computers alike. If this happens, data may be destroyed. Procedures must be established for protecting these data (medical records, personnel files, accounts receivable, and so forth) and for operating in a manual mode in the event full computer operations cannot be continued.
- Is there a specific written list of roles and responsibilities for personnel serving in the Command Post? Is there an identical list available for the Personnel Pool to provide for appropriate assignment of support personnel to the Command Post?
- Are procedures written to detail procurement of needed supplies/equipment for areas requesting support? Is there a priority system for decisions regarding

which areas will receive their orders when supplies/equipment become limited? Have arrangements been made with outside vendors, including suppliers of equipment, bottled water, pharmaceuticals, and whole blood/blood products, for additional supplies when inhouse resources drop below acceptable amounts? Have "acceptable amounts" (par levels) been determined?

1. Opening the Command Post

Because the Command Post is the vital link between facility units and the procurement of additional supplies/equipment and personnel, and between the internal operations of the facility and the outside response system, this area must function with a high degree of efficiency and integrity. The Command Post is one unit that will not be able to improvise and still maintain adequate control. All aspects of its operation require careful thought and detailing before a disaster.

The Command Post is the central unit for managing response. Adequate recordkeeping is imperative. Exhibit 4–10 is an example of a master Command Post status control document.

If the facility is an acute care hospital with a 24-hour emergency department, the ED may want to establish its own Command Post in or near that unit. From this location the ED administrators can, with clerical and messenger support, provide a communication link to the hospital Command Post. A good deal of information moves into an ED mobilized for a disaster. This information needs to be integrated and forwarded to facility administration rapidly. In addition, the ED interfaces with organized emergency response teams in the field and generally is aware immediately of status changes in an external disaster. Finally, Triage and the Major Treatment Area are located within the jurisdiction of the ED and require careful administrative tracking and control to prevent loss of continuity of care, queuing, and further staff/equipment/supply overload problems.

2. Staffing and Equipment

Whether it is a facilitywide Command Post or the ED's Command Post, personnel assignments and responsibilities, communication equipment, operational supplies/equipment, and operational procedures for that area must be developed carefully and included in the ED subsection of the *Disaster Manual*.

Section IV Personnel Pool

This part of the manual on managing the allocation of personnel should detail:

1. Function
2. Staffing and Equipment
3. Procedures.

Exhibit 4-10 Example of Hospital Command Post Personnel Status Form

Date: _____
Disaster Onset Date: _____

Station	Time of Logging	Total RNs	Total LVNs	Total MDs	Total Clerks	Total Messengers	Total Techs	Problems/Notes
Triage Area								
Major Treatment								
Delayed Care								
Surgery								
ICU								
Lab								
Radiology								
Medical Unit, 2nd floor								
Surgical Unit, 3rd floor								

Totals to Date:

Casualties Triaged _____   DOA _____   Transferred _____
        Admitted _____   Expired in-house _____

1. Function

Exhibit 4–11 is an example of a Personnel Pool operations procedure. The Personnel Pool is responsible for the following tasks:

- Identifying positively all health personnel arriving at the pool location
- Providing identifying insignia or apparel to all arriving personnel
- Allocating personnel based upon specifications set forth in the plan
- Documenting personnel actions

2. Staffing and Equipment

The personnel needs of individual departments must be defined. This assures that departments and units will be sent someone who is reasonably capable of

---

Exhibit 4–11 Example of Personnel Pool Operations Procedure

Function of Personnel Pool

1. Maintains records of personnel work times and assignments
2. Processes incoming personnel
3. Allocates resources as requested by units and according to specifications

Staffing Personnel Pool

1. One director
2. Two or more messengers
3. Two or more clerks

Staff Classification	Assignment
Clerk(s)	1. Check ID of all incoming personnel
	2. Document arrivals, using staff resources form
	3. Direct arriving personnel to a hold area
	4. Document who is sent where, and when
	5. Forward staffing data to the Command Post every hour
Director, Personnel Pool	1. Receive staff requests from units
	2. Select personnel for assignment based upon specifications (classifications and experience) for each unit
	3. Dispatch personnel to requesting units
Messenger(s)	1. Deliver documents to designated areas
	2. Return promptly to Personnel Pool

providing the assistance needed. Examples of specifications for Triage personnel are:

- Triage Area Medical Officer

    a. MD, specializing in emergency medicine
    b. May be an RN credentialed in advanced cardiac life support (ACLS) and emergency nursing, with recent clinical experience in emergency services and in triage of emergency patients

- Triage RN

    a. Experienced in emergency services, with recent clinical experience
    b. Trained in physical assessment of trauma victims

- Triage LVN or Emergency Care Technician
    a. LVN with experience in emergency care, or
    b. EMT-A with experience and training in physical assessment, or
    c. ECT with six months' experience in an ED

- Clerk

    a. Lay person with ability to speak English, coordinate statistics, and maintain a flow log

- Transporter

    a. Lay person without physical handicap
    b. Able to speak English and follow directions efficiently

3. Procedures

Procedures for allocating personnel resources must be clearly stated and detailed in the Personnel Pool section of the manual.

Section V Communications

The manual section labeled Communications should contain sections on:

1. Function
2. Staffing and Equipment
3. Procedures.

1. Function

Communication systems consist of hardware (such as telephone and computer equipment) and software (computer instructions and disks, and procedure manuals, including the *Disaster Manual*). Communication breakdown is one of the most common problems in disaster situations. Telephones become overloaded or nonfunctional, paper work is easily lost and often is poorly documented, and messengers sometimes are unavailable because they become lost, are given other tasks, or their assignment to appropriate departments or areas does not occur. Alternative resources for communications, should breakdowns occur, must be established well before they are needed.

2. Staffing and Equipment

The following questions should be addressed in preparing this subsection:

- Is the institution equipped with a two-way radio to maintain communications with outside agencies, other facilities, and ground units if such units are likely to deliver patients to the facility?
- Have procedures been defined for locating and securing pay telephones if they will be used to supplement or back up the hospital switchboard? How are sufficient coins for their use to be made available?
- Have emergency communication links been established with:

    a. adjacent hospitals and SNFs
    b. law enforcement agencies
    c. fire authorities
    d. water, gas, hazardous waste collection companies
    e. community resources that will supply the facility with extra food, water, supplies, equipment
    f. community resources such as Civil Defense, Salvation Army, American Red Cross, local ham radio operators
    g. the county disaster coordination center.

- Has someone been made responsible for securing telephone communications?

The assurance of telephone operations may require extensive predisaster consultation with the telephone company and with equipment vendors. A telephone system, while vulnerable to events that down lines, can be hardened for situations such as overload (i.e., too many incoming and outgoing calls). Someone also must be designated the responsibility for ensuring continuity of two-way radio operations. Because the time at which disaster occurs is not predictable, several persons, preferably one for each shift, should be trained in the use of all radio equipment that will operate during such an event.

3. Procedures

Procedures that prescribe the use of intrafacility communication systems must be developed. These should include procedures for two-way, hand-held radio and direct-line telephone operations, and backup procedures for checking equipment function when stored and not in use.

Procedures must be developed that specify messenger assignment, training, and use of identification insignia.

Examples of paper work requirements should be included in this section as well.

Section VI Paper Work and Forms

This section of the manual should specify forms and include completed samples.

A disaster disrupts routine and causes confusion and chaos. Adequate documentation, however, can markedly mitigate the disruption. Proper documentation is essential to evaluate response and to recover costs. Working forms must be stored in the response areas. Samples are presented in Appendix 4–C at the end of this chapter (and are discussed next).

Disaster Tag

Regardless of whether field personnel initially conduct triage and tag casualties, the receiving facility must have sufficient tags available for retagging. Triage is always a continuum, since emergency patients and disaster casualties are dynamic until proven stable. Retriage at the hospital may reveal that a victim's status has changed significantly; hospital tags can be placed on the patient's arm along with the field tag to indicate the retriage priority, even if it remains the same priority as that determined in the field. Field tags may provide sufficient information for field teams to identify priorities for transport, but hospitals generally require more specific information regarding initial stabilization as well as disposition within the facility. Field tags also may become unreadable or detached. Therefore, facilities often choose to apply their own tags when victims arrive.

Depending on how fast and in what numbers casualties are received, the ED or other receiving area will not have time to generate a patient record. The facility tag may have to substitute for a chart, perhaps for some time, and should be compact and capable of being recorded in duplicate. The tag remains with the patient while the copy is forwarded to the facility Command Post as an admitting document and as a record from which to tabulate volume and cost estimates subsequent to the event. (See Appendix 4–C, Exhibit A.)

Triage Casualty Log

Since triage is a serial process, Triage Casualty Logs should be located at *each area* in the facility receiving patients from ED triage to document who was received, the time of arrival, the tag number, triage priority, and the time the victim left ED triage. Regardless of the receiving department/area, disaster casualties should not be mixed with the general patient register unless some specific method is used to provide for rapid retrieval of casualty information. The Triage Area Casualty Log for the triage area must identify all incoming victims, arrival times, tag numbers, the disposition of victims, and time out of triage. (See Appendix 4–C, Exhibit B.)

Casualty Disposition Log

This log would be helpful in large institutions with several exits to inpatient areas from the Triage Area. Even though the Triage Area Casualty Log specifies disposition and time out, patients may become lost within the facility unless workers stationed at exits document who left, where they were going, who was transporting them, their tag numbers, and departure times. The Casualty Disposition Log is an additional safety check for tracking purposes (Appendix 4–C, Exhibit C).

Disaster Initial Notification Form

Whoever receives initial notification is required to complete this form because it provides baseline information about the event. Decisions on implementation of disaster response are based on this information, and on 15- and 30-minute update forms completed subsequently. The Disaster Initial Notification Form is available from local hospital councils or disaster planning agencies or can be developed by the facility. (See Exhibit 4–6, above.)

Hourly Individual Area Status Report Form

Because initial information regarding the event may be revised significantly as further details are obtained from the field, hourly status reports are used to document changes affecting facility capability. These forms should include information needed for decision making while mobilization continues (Appendix 4–C, Exhibit D).

Implementation Status Form

This form is used to document action taken by individuals responsible for mobilizing an area, or even the entire facility. It also is used for response critique and follow-up. For this reason, actions taken, and the time, must be noted. While only brief, concise, and essential actions should be cited, the report form could total as many as three to five pages (Appendix 4–C, Exhibit E).

Departmental Critique Form

Each mobilizing department/area should be able to track events for later critique. The form can be modified to meet differing department needs. (See Appendix 5–B at the end of Chapter 5.)

Personnel Assignment Form

While service areas may want to use a blackboard system for documenting assignments, a Personnel Assignment Form can be very helpful to Command Post and Personnel Pool administrators. This form documents both the assignments and the number and duration of rest breaks. In disasters of long duration, administration will need a way to monitor hours of duty to ensure that personnel do not work excessively without rest breaks. (See Appendix 4–C, Exhibit F.)

Callback Lists

As discussed earlier, these lists should be prepared in duplicate so that a copy can be forwarded to the Command Post.

Area Disaster Personnel/Supplies/Equipment Form

Disasters can exhaust on-hand supplies quickly. This form is used to request equipment and supplies, to document the need for reorders, and to aid Command Post personnel in apportioning resources if need be. The form identifies other aspects of department status, as well, and serves to keep the Command Post aware of factors such as the number of personnel on site, evacuation activity, etc. (See Appendix 4–C, Exhibit G.)

Disaster Action Cards

Because true disaster situations are unpredictable and extremely variable, drills alone will not prepare personnel for optimum functioning in every specific circumstance. Staff turnover, excitement, anxiety, and a feeling of urgency or haste can confuse even experienced personnel. Roles are easily forgotten in the urgency of the moment. Disaster Action Cards are a simple method for assigning and identifying roles and responsibilities for all personnel. (Exhibit 4–12 provides two examples.)

No one will have time during a disaster to reread the manual for directions. But those involved do need to know what is expected of them. Issuing every assigned staff member and physician a card that, point by point, defines no more than seven

Exhibit 4-12 Examples of Disaster Action Cards

Front of Card

ED CLERK

Front of Card

ED CHARGE NURSE

ED Clerk

1. Notify X-ray at extension xxx.
2. Notify lab at extension yyy.
3. Notify ED physicians with direction from doctor on duty.
4. Notify ED administrators with direction from nurse in charge.
5. Begin staff call-in until relieved by ED Command Post; obtain direction as necessary from nurse in charge.
6. Refer all public inquiries to hospital administration at extension zzz.
7. Proceed to Triage Area to assist in tagging victims relieved by assigned personnel.

Back of Card

ED Charge Nurse

1. Notify ED physician and share all available information.
2. Call Nursing Supervisor at extension 000 or page
   a. advise of extent and type of disaster
   b. request immediate response to ED to help
3. Survey department for available treatment areas; help determine which patients can be discharged, admitted, or transferred.
4. Assign triage nurse and technician; hand out cards.
5. Assign one critical care team; hand out cards.
6. Assign staff to ED and delayed treatment areas; hand out cards.
7. Assume responsibility for nursing disaster coordination until relieved by ED nursing supervisor or assistant.
8. Notify waiting room patients of situation.
9. Assign arriving staff to patient care responsibilities.

Back of Card

Source: Reprinted from ''Disaster Management'' by J.K. Simoneau in *Emergency Nursing: Principles and Practice*, 2nd ed., S.A. Sheehy and J.M. Barber (Eds.), with permission of the C.V. Mosby Company, St. Louis, © 1985.

necessary actions to take immediately and in order of priority makes appropriate response more certain. (See additional examples in Appendix 4–C, Exhibit H.)

Because they must be working documents, Disaster Action Cards should be laminated with clear material to prevent destruction from moisture or soilage. Copies should be maintained in the Disaster Supply cupboard of each area and the originals kept in a safe and clean location for reproduction later as needed. Because the working copies may be either lost or damaged beyond repair, copies can be made from the originals and replaced immediately in the supply cupboard. Telephone extensions and the names of specific persons who must be contacted by specific individuals should be printed on appropriate cards and updated periodically.

Section VII Triage Area

This section of the manual has three subsections:

1. Function
2. Staffing and Equipment
3. Procedures.

The term "triage" derives from the French verb "trier," meaning "to sort," and the French noun "triage," meaning "sorting," "selection," "classification." The process of triage in a disaster is serial, with retriage occurring at each point of receipt of casualties: transportation to facility, at the facility Triage Area, and at individual receiving units. The manual must designate a Triage Area. Generally it should be near the ED, although the location should not be finalized until the facility's traffic and evacuation route patterns have been analyzed.

The Triage Area and ED are not the same units. The former operates only when the Triage Code has been declared. Its role is the rapid evaluation and assignment of patients. The ED function, on the other hand, is to stabilize only those with life-threatening injuries. When the facility can expect to receive more than ten victims from a disaster incident, the Triage Area should be opened to accommodate flow and serve as a barrier to the curious. Only life-saving care and minimal attempts to cover wounds should occur in this area. If more is attempted, queuing will result and necessitate additional clinical personnel in the area.

Usually external triage and tagging will have been performed by public safety personnel before victims reach the institution. However, mass casualty situations may generate so many victims that sorting and tagging in the field is hasty, sporadic, and may have a high classification error rate. Tags may be missing, torn, or bloody. Status changes may have occurred en route that result in classification differences when the patients arrive. It thus is best that each victim be reevaluated rapidly and retagged to prevent distribution and management errors in the facility. The classification system used by an institution can be either its own or one prescribed by regional disaster planning agencies. (See Appendix 4–D for common systems of triage.)

Ideally, the Triage Area should be located adjacent to the ED. If there is no ED, then Triage should be next to the area designated to evaluate and stabilize life-threatening and critical cases. Several other physical considerations must be taken into account when determining the best location for Triage. The area should be:

- under a roof or canopy that will shield victims and personnel from inclement weather
- accessible to rescue vehicles directly
- accessible to irrigation/shower equipment for radiation and hazardous chemical contamination cases
- equipped with appropriate lighting or able to accommodate supplemental lighting
- securable, with only limited access by nonauthorized persons
- located so that victims can be referred easily to all of the likely receiving units in the facility
- accessible to the morgue or designated temporary morgue.

Protection from adverse weather is important. Triage Area personnel will not be able to work in adverse conditions very long, and victims should be shielded from exposure if at all possible. Accessibility for ambulance traffic is vital. Impediments to the forward flow of traffic produce delays in depositing victims and returning to the field. If the traffic flow is forward (one-way) only, chances for collision are minimized. If the facility has a parking lot access gate that will delay movement of rescue vehicles, someone must be responsible for ensuring that the control arm is locked in the "up" position. A security officer should be stationed there to prevent others from using or blocking the gate.

Security of the Triage Area is a must. Unauthorized persons can hinder its function and detract from the privacy that victims must be afforded, particularly from the news media. While hospital entrances must be locked and guarded to prevent injured walk-ins and public from entering the facility unnoticed, one alternate entrance should be designated for arriving personnel so that the Triage Area is not used as a passageway. The public can be routed through one guarded and specifically identified entrance that is not in the Triage Area. However, walk-in victims should be encouraged to enter through the Triage Area so they can be evaluated in the same manner as other casualties.

1. Function

The primary function of a disaster Triage Area is a rapid assessment of all incoming casualties, the assignment of priorities for management, and classification of dispositions. Without a Triage Area to manage the patient flow, the Major Treatment Area may become overwhelmed.

2. Staffing and Equipment

Personnel assigned to the Triage Area include message runners, transporters, clerical staff, nurses, and physicians. One person (the Triage Medical Officer) should have overall responsibility for coordination. The number of persons assigned to Triage varies. However, minimal staffing for a general acute care hospital or larger SNF is:

- one MD skilled in triage
- one RN skilled in triage
- one LVN or Emergency Care Technician
- one clerk
- six transporters
- two message runners

If a physician is not available, an RN with training in the concepts of casualty triage and emergency patient assessment can be designated as the triage officer. Emergency Department nurses are appropriate substitutes if they have had triage experience. Whoever is assigned to the role must be able to perform rapid assessments, make rapid triage decisions with a high rate of precision, understand disaster triage and have a high tolerance for stress. Any triage officer must abandon traditional concepts of total patient care and accept instead the disaster need for rapid evaluation/distribution of victims. A rule of thumb in assigning sufficient personnel is the following:

- one triage officer can see one or two victims per minute, for brief bursts of influx (occasionally a patient may take three to five minutes)
- more than 30 patients per hour will require a second triager and a sufficient number of taggers to prevent delay.[3]

The LVN/ECT role is to complete tags, attach them to victims, and retrieve valuables and clothing for bagging. The clerk tags the bag and completes the Triage Area Casualty Log.

All personnel assigned must remain in the Triage Area until either the disaster is officially declared over or relief personnel arrive. Provisions must be made to allow sufficient rest breaks if the disaster is prolonged.

All personnel assigned to the Triage Area must understand the system of classification being used. Transporters must be thoroughly familiar with the patient flow pattern and locations for distribution. Signs also should be posted to designate these areas. A location board identifying access routes to areas designated as receiving units for casualties may prove helpful when many transporters are used or when volunteers are used who are unfamiliar with the locations. In addition, at least one security officer should be stationed in the Triage Area to direct families, sightseers, news media, blood donors, etc., who come to the area. Figure 4–3 depicts triaged casualty flow in a typical acute care hospital.

Only limited but totally dedicated hospital supplies should be located in the Triage Area. A triage cart should be kept stocked and stored near the site. The following supplies are suggested:

- disaster tags
- Triage Area Casualty Log
- clipboards, pencils, pens
- marking pens
- bullhorn and/or two-way radios
- supply cart
- laundry cart with hamper bag
- portable suction unit
- E-cylinder oxygen tanks
- ambu bags with assorted mask sizes
- aromatic ammonia capsules
- clothing bags
- blankets
- penlights
- plastic IV solution bags to use as replacement bags for solution infused or nearly empty on arrival
- OB delivery packs
- arm and leg splints and splint padding
- sterile gauze 4/4 pads
- rubber oral airways, all sizes
- bag/valve resuscitator bag.

Figure 4–3 Example of Hospital Triage Flow

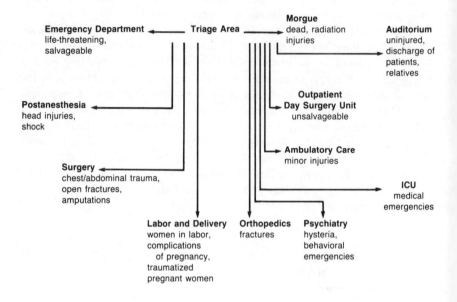

Provisions must be made for immediate delivery of sufficient wheelchairs, gurneys, sheets, and IV poles upon opening of the Triage Area in an actual disaster.

One frequently overlooked element is the supply needs of incoming ambulances. Attendants will not be able to return to quarters to resupply before returning to the field for more victims. If the disaster is of significant magnitude, arrangements should be made to provide them with resupply packs containing items most often used in a disaster: sterile dressing and bandage supplies, splinting materials, plastic IV bags, airway equipment, and oxygen administration sets. Prior coordination with local providers of rescue services to determine the precise compilation of these "readi-paks" is essential.

Provision also must be made for Central Service to replace used Triage supplies immediately. This can be accomplished most easily by stationing a Central Service staff member at Triage with a simple inventory list. Runners are used to obtain additional supplies as needed. Where Central Service and the facility are not large enough to permit this, another procedure must be developed to ensure resupply on another basis.

Exhibit 4–13 Example of Tagging Procedure for Triage Area

---

1. All patients are expected to arrive from the field with a Disaster Tag tied to one of their limbs. Attach a hospital tag to the same extremity. Do not remove the field tag.
2. The Triage Area clerk should attempt to fill in the victim's *name, date, time, age,* and *sex* on the hospital tag as rapidly as possible.
3. The portion of the tag labeled "Medical" should be filled out by the triage officer or assistant.
4. "Initial routing directions" should designate

    a. major treatment
    b. minor treatment or
    c. morgue

    according to the instructions of the triage officer.

5. The pull-off, self-adhesive, numbered stickers from the reverse side of the tag should be placed on the Triage Casualty Log. (If possible, put the patient's name by the number.)
6. The Triage Casualty Log must include:

    a. the victim's numbered sticker (name if possible)
    b. time of victim's arrival
    c. destination

        • major treatment
        • minor treatment
        • morgue

    d. time out.

---

3. Procedures

Procedures should prescribe expectations for individual and organizational unit responses. Exhibit 4–13 is an example of typical instruction (in this case for Triage Area tagging) in this subsection of the manual. Examples of other necessary procedures statements for this subsection are included as Exhibits 4–14, 4–15, and 4–16.

Figure 4–4 is a flow chart outlining the steps Triage workers can follow in assessing casualties.

Because of the importance of triage, several questions should be answered before assembling final materials for the Triage Area section of the manual:

• Have both the location and an alternate site been designated and is a layout drawing available for inclusion in the manual?

Exhibit 4–14 Example of General Procedures Statement for the Triage Area

1. Do not remove casualties from the litters on which they are brought to the area.
2. Evaluate the airway, breathing, and circulation (ABCs) rapidly:

   - patency of the airway
   - adequacy of ventilations: rate, rhythm, depth, symmetry of chest rise, lung sounds
   - adequacy of circulation: external bleeding, all peripheral pulses and their quality, rate, rhythm
   - condition of the cervical spine: tenderness, pain, paresthesias, paralysis.

3. Assess all injuries by performing a rapid head-to-toe evaluation using the techniques of inspection, palpation, and auscultation.
4. Assign a treatment priority and disposition.
5. *Talk to* and reassure all victims.

- If outside, have weather protection, lighting, security, privacy been addressed?
- Is the area accessible by rescue vehicles?
- How will Triage personnel be identified (i.e., pullover smocks, bibs, armbands)?
- Have procedures been explained regarding linkage and communication between the Triage Area and the receiving areas?
- Have Disaster Action Cards been prepared for each staff member/category assigned to Triage?
- Has a disaster supply cart been stocked and are ambulance resupply packs stored in close proximity to the Triage Area?
- Is there a procedure for periodic inventory of ambulance resupply packs and for inventory during a disaster?

Exhibit 4–15 Example of Triage Patient Flow Procedures

1. Do not attempt to provide patient care.
2. Area availability for disposition will be identified by the triage officer.
3. Queuing must be prevented in the Triage Area. If it begins, request assistance from the ED Command Post.
4. All casualties arriving in, and leaving, the Triage Area must be logged in on the Casualty Log.

Exhibit 4–16 Example of Triage Rating System

Five-tier system (used in military triage)
Dead or will die
Life-threatening—readily correctable
Urgent—must be treated within one to two hours
Delayed—noncritical or ambulatory
No injury—no treatment necessary

Four-tier system
Immediate—seriously injured, reasonable chance of survival
Delayed—can wait for care after simple first aid
Expectant—extremely critical, moribund
Minimal—no impairment of function, can either treat self or be treated by a nonprofessional

Three-tier system
Life-threatening—readily correctable
Urgent—must be treated within one to two hours
Delayed—no injury, noncritical, or ambulatory

Two-tier system
Immediate versus delayed:
    Immediate—life-threatening injuries that are readily correctable on scene, and those that
      are urgent
    Delayed—no injury, noncritical injuries, ambulatory victims, moribund, and dead

Source: Reprinted from "Disaster Management" by J.K. Simoneau, in *Emergency Nursing: Principles and Practice,* 2nd ed., S.A. Sheehy and J.M. Barber (Eds.), with permission of the C.V. Mosby Company, St. Louis, © 1985.

- Has a disaster traffic flow pattern been developed to accommodate arriving personnel, walk-in patients, forward flow of casualties from Triage, and paper work?
- Has a classification system for victims been established in conjunction with disaster agency personnel, field personnel, and adjacent facilities, as appropriate?
- Have policies/procedures been developed for the:

—assessment process
—documentation process
—distribution process
—extent of stabilization
—procurement of supplies
—traffic flow
—disposition of dead/will die victims
—handling of clothing and valuables.

Figure 4–4 Sample Triage and Rapid Treatment Diagram

START

Simple Triage and Rapid Treatment

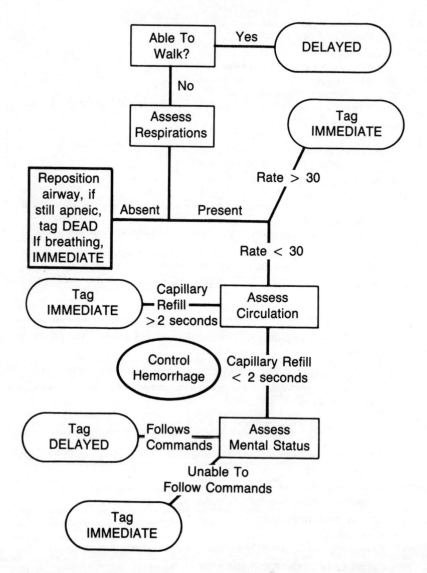

Source: Reprinted with permission from *Paramedic*, Vol. 6, No. 1, p. 14, © January-February 1985.

Section VIII Major Treatment Area

This section of the manual has three subsections:

1. Function
2. Staffing and Equipment
3. Procedures.

The types and number of actual "treating" areas that will receive casualties from the Triage Area vary from facility to facility. These areas should be designated based on the categories of victims the institution may reasonably expect to receive. For instance, in a controlled distribution, a skilled nursing facility would be most likely to receive evacuated inpatients from acute care hospitals seeking to make room for casualty intake. The evacuated patients should be sorted into groups (i.e., medical, surgical, isolation, etc.) and be distributed within the facility appropriately.

Acute care hospitals receiving life-threatening, urgent, and delayed cases will have to determine which areas are appropriate, both logistically and clinically, for casualty care. That determination will depend upon the size of the facility and the types of inpatient services available on a daily basis. An example of the possibilities follows

Emergency Department: All life-threatening categories; all victims requiring initiation of IV lines; chemical ocular injuries

Surgery: Penetrating abdominal/chest trauma; extensive lacerations/avulsions; traumatic eye injuries; amputations; blunt abdominal trauma with hemodynamic compromise; multisystem trauma

Surgical ICU: Head injury with altered level of consciousness; postarrest victims; moderate burns; blunt abdominal trauma with equivocal signs

Recovery Room: Serious burns; fractures requiring operative repair; extensive lacerations/abrasions

Medical ICU: Blunt chest trauma; r/o acute myocardial infarction (MI); nontraumatic respiratory distress; smoke inhalation

Clinic Auditorium: Strains/sprains; simple lacerations; minor head trauma; minor surface trauma; minor first degree and second degree burns

Chapel: Emotional/psychological disturbances, if nonviolent

Psychiatry: Violent behavior

Morgue: Victims without vital signs if no life support estab-
                         lished in field; injuries obviously incompatible with
                         resuscitation (decapitation, amputation of two or
                         more extremities and no life signs, rigor mortis, etc.)

The point to be borne in mind is to avoid relocating the disaster from the field to facility treatment areas. If at all possible, the casualties should be distributed such that no one area is inundated significantly. If the disaster is large, producing tremendous numbers of victims, hospitals in and adjacent to the impact area would soon become overwhelmed. In such an eventuality, the region and/or state and/or the federal government would mobilize mutual aid. For the more common multiple casualty incidents, however, it is possible to determine which areas are suitable for which types of victims, and how those areas should be staffed. Improper, uncoordinated, and uncontrolled distribution of casualties received is a major intrahospital problem and should be addressed by disaster planners. Questions to be raised in preparing this section of the manual are:

- Which areas will receive casualties, based on the triage categories established by the facility?
- Has a system been developed to identify which victims will go where from the Triage Area?
- Who will staff these areas? Will personnel from the Emergency Department be needed anywhere other than in the ED? (Some facilities send one or two clinical staff members from the ED to the Delayed Care Area.)
- What personnel specifications would the Personnel Pool use to obtain further staffing when an area becomes overloaded?
- Who will have the authority to deter the Triage Area from sending further victims into an overwhelmed unit? How will this be accomplished? Where else will incoming victims in that category be sent?
- What equipment/supplies will be needed to meet the needs of casualties and staff?
- Who will have the responsibility for developing Disaster Action Cards for personnel assigned in each of the treatment areas?
- Has an efficient system been established to ensure sufficient numbers of physicians for each treatment area (except the morgue)?

1. Function

Figure 4–3 (earlier) depicts the patient flow to the Major Treatment Area and other areas in a typical acute care hospital. Such a diagram would be an appropriate insert for this subsection of the manual. The function of the Major Treatment Area is to process casualties with life-threatening injuries and provide initial evaluation and stabilization (airways, IVs, chest tubes, etc.) before transfer to other definitive care areas.

2. Staffing and Equipment

Materials describing personnel responsibilities for the Major Treatment Area should be included in this subsection.

Some facilities operate this area using the critical care team concept. This concept was developed out of a need to provide for continuity of care under Emergency Department overload situations. Fragmentation of both medical attention and nursing care is highly likely when there are numbers of seriously or critically injured victims and insufficient staff to attend them. It can be assumed that victims classified as "immediate" will require 1:1 nursing care and efficient and continuous medical and nursing intervention. In cases where the ED is able to limit the number of "immediate" cases, one patient is assigned to a single critical care team. The first team can be drawn from staff already in the department. As more personnel arrive, more teams can be assembled. In fact, staffing needs for call-back can be more easily identified if critical care teams are used, since the number of teams needed dictates the number and type of staffing necessary. For maximum effectiveness, each team should consist of the following members:

- a physician experienced in emergency care
- an emergency nurse
- an emergency care technician (ECT)
- a clerk.

The success of the operation depends on how quickly the teams can be established, how well they understand their role, and how effectively the members remain together and work as a team. The role of each team, which may be designated as Team 1, Team 2, etc., is to accept a patient in the ED from the Triage Area, perform appropriate and reasonable life-saving intervention, and admit the victim either to an operating room or a critical care unit for further stabilization. The patient classified as "immediate" should remain in the ED for as brief a period as possible.

All members of a critical care team together should transport the victim to the appropriate in-hospital area, then return to the ED for immediate reassignment of another patient. In the case of a mass casualty disaster where the number of "immediate" priority cases exceeds the department's ability to provide enough teams, the teams may have to provide care for more than one victim at a time. However, their purpose will be negated if they attempt to manage more than two cases at the same time.

Several important factors can contribute to the effectiveness of these teams:

- A critical care team must remain together until the disaster is resolved and no further receipt of casualties is expected. The teams should not disband until the Disaster Coordinator advises them that the disaster operation has been declared over and no further patients are being processed from the field.
- A team should manage its patient as quickly as possible by evaluating priorities of treatment as a unit, providing the treatment necessary to stabilize the patient, then transferring the victim to a definitive care area. This assures continuity of care and the provision of a patient care report directly to the receiving unit staff.
- Once a victim has been evaluated and transferred, the team should reassemble for assignment of another case immediately.
- A team should be identified by letter or number, and each member should wear an identifying armband or bib stating Team A or Team 1, etc.
- Physicians from the medical staff who are used must be willing to remain on their teams until relieved by another MD and not take victims as their own patients, thereby leaving teams without a physician.

The physician member generates the medical treatment orders and serves as principal clinician. In the event a physician is not available to head the team, experienced emergency nurses have been used with success in this role. The RN provides emergency intervention and documents treatment. The ECT provides equipment and supplies and assists the nurse and physician. The clerk prepares clothing and valuables lists, bags clothing, completes stat lab and urgent X-ray requisitions, and makes certain that a chart is generated for the patient, the Disaster Distribution Log is filled out, and that disposition of the Disaster Tag soft copy is appropriate.

3. Procedures

This subsection should detail all appropriate casualty management procedures. Exhibit 4–17 is an example of a procedure statement for handling a casualty.

Exhibit 4–17 Example of a Major Treatment Area Procedure for Handling a Casualty Death after Admission

1. Include a copy of the treatment record and/or disaster tag with the body when it is sent to the morgue.
2. Cover the body with a clean sheet for transport to the morgue.
3. Tie a patient ID tag on the left great toe. If that toe is not intact, place the tag on an intact extremity digit.
4. Log the casualty disposition on the area log.
5. Send clothing and valuables with the body to the morgue.
6. Refer all calls and messages regarding the case to the Hospital Command Post.
7. Direct family and friends to the chaplain's office, accompanied by a staff member.

Section IX Delayed Care Area

This section of the manual defines the role of the Delayed Care Area and includes three subsections:

1. Function
2. Staffing and Equipment
3. Procedures.

1. Function

The function of this area is to receive, evaluate, treat as necessary, and provide disposition for all casualties without serious or life-threatening injuries. Because this may involve a large number of casualties, the Delayed Care Area should be in a location capable of accommodating large numbers.

2. Staffing and Equipment

Staffing should include one surgeon or emergency physician, one or two RNs (preferably emergency nurses) and several experienced medical/surgical nurses. Clerks, messengers, and transporters can be obtained from the Personnel Pool as needed. Equipment should include gurneys, liners, bandaging supplies, basins, antiseptic solutions, casting materials, etc.

3. Procedures

This section should contain written procedures for patient care, treatment systems, and procedures for disposition of patients.

Section X Departmental Responsibilities

This section is designed to assure coordinated response throughout the institution. The same format should be used for each department's process. The procedures should be included in the manual and duplicated, and distributed as minimanuals to each department as well. Exhibits 4–18, 4–19, and 4–20 give examples for treatment, service, and administrative departments.

Ancillary Service departments such as housekeeping, food services, plant engineering, and so forth, face unusual demands in a disaster. They often are looked to for "extra" personnel to perform roles such as messenger and security, yet must maintain their own service function at the same time. Questions to consider in preparing procedures for these departments include:

- Is an outside vendor (e.g., laboratory, laundry, blood bank) expected to supplement the facility's own supplies? If so, has an updated vendor list been compiled?
- Have policies been established to define and resolve additional staffing needs?

Exhibit 4–18 Example of Surgical Department Disaster Manual Procedure

DEPARTMENT OF SURGERY

Surgical Supervisor
Alternate: Assistant Supervisor

Procedure for Code Triage Full Operation:

1. Cancel scheduled elective surgeries.

2. Prepare all rooms for emergency surgeries.

3. Request all additional help from Personnel Pool.

4. Request supplies, as needed, from Central Service.

5. Make the medical personnel pool responsible for physician assignments in each operating suite.

6. Preoperative orders may be carried out in Surgery:
   a. Check reverse side of original copy of victim Disaster Tag for:
      (1) physician orders
      (2) medications and time given.

7. After surgery is complete, call Admitting for room assignment.

8. Follow disposition of personal effects and valuables.

Exhibit 4–19 Example of Ancillary Department Disaster Manual Procedure

---

LAUNDRY

Director of Laundry Services
Alternate: Assistant Laundry Manager

Procedure for Code Triage Full Operation:

All on-duty laundry service personnel will report to the Laundry. Personnel called to the hospital will report to the Personnel Pool located in the North Building.

The Laundry Department will:

1. Provide extra linen as ordered to casualty treatment areas
2. Dispatch a laundry cart with linen and blankets to the Triage Area
3. Pick up and deliver linens to casualty treatment areas
4. Put laundry operations on a 24-hour schedule for duration of emergency
5. Order additional linen as needed.

The following items will be delivered immediately to the casualty areas indicated:

Morgue	20 each:	Sheets
		Towels
		Washclothes
Delayed Care Area	50 each:	Blankets
		Gowns
		Sheets
		Towels
		Washcloths
Major Treatment Area	20 each:	Blankets
		Gowns
		Sheets
		Towels
		Washcloths
Other Areas:	On standby for calls as needed.	

- Is any ancillary service department expected to provide personnel for other disaster support tasks? If so, are there specific procedures for establishing need, allocating personnel, and providing coverage (i.e., housekeepers performing as transporters, language interpreters)?
- Does each service area have the supplies and equipment it will need to provide disaster support? How will additional pharmaceutical supplies be obtained when the existing materials are exhausted?
- Have arrangements been made for additional food and water supplies?

Exhibit 4–20 Example of Administrative Department Disaster Manual
Procedure

MEDICAL RECORDS/ACCOUNTING

Director of Medical Records
Alternate: Supervisor, Medical Records

Procedure for Code Triage Full Operation:

1. The director or designee will assign one person to go immediately to the Emergency Department and one to the Delayed Care Area to report to the person in charge of each area and to assist with compilation of medical record information.
2. The director or designee will provide direction for employees and personnel assigned from the Personnel Pool in the identification and registration of casualties and the generation of treatment records.
3. Admitting clerks on the 3-11 or 11-7 shifts will notify Director of Medical Records or alternate of the emergency and, at their direction, implement Disaster Callback procedure.
4. Prepared packets are available in the Emergency Department that contain treatment records with assigned pseudo numbers. These pseudo numbers are never to be changed and will constitute the patient's permanent ID number.
5. Disaster Tags placed in the field are to remain on patients until final disposition, even if the Triage Area retags the victims.
6. A messenger from Medical Records/Accounting must pick up medical records hourly from these treatment areas:

   Major Treatment—Emergency Department
   Neurology: Initial treatment—South Corridor
   Psychiatric: Initial treatment—North Corridor
   Cardiopulmonary: Initial treatment—Benson Lobby
   Abdominal: Initial treatment—West Corridor
   Burn: Initial treatment—East Corridor Door A
   Orthopedic: Initial treatment—Outpatient Patio
   Triage: Triage Area
   Morgue: Morgue and Elm Street garage annex.

- Have procedures been set up for equipment repair, disbursement, and procurement for the Purchasing Department?

The same types of questions may be applied to administrative departments as well. Exhibit 4–20 is an example of a procedure for a Medical Records Department.

Facility security is a vital element in a disaster situation. The facility plan and the manual must provide direction to the Security force for managing both internal and external disasters. Many institutions do not have a substantial Security force and will need to identify carefully appropriate surrogates to undertake the responsibility of Security. Controlling access routes into the institution, identification of authorized personnel, direction control and information delivery, and management of disruptive citizens are aspects requiring consideration. When determining what elements of the facility plan need to be developed or revised in this section, the following should be considered:

- How will authorized staff entering the facility be identified? How will mutual aid responders sent to augment staff be identified? (It may be necessary to work with local disaster agency planners to establish this aspect.)
- Which entries will be designated for news media and community agency personnel (i.e., Red Cross, blood bank services, etc.)?
- Is there a registration system to track all nonemployees? Will it use a sign-in system, dispense badges, etc.?
- How will Security officers be identified? Uniforms will be more effective than plain clothes. How will uniforms be distributed for surrogates designated to perform Security roles?
- Is there a policy and procedure for the immediate securing of all facility access routes upon notification of a disaster?
- Is there a system to prevent entry into restricted areas of the facility by unauthorized personnel/persons?
- Are there specific procedures for coping with acts of terrorism?
- Are there procedures for notification of local law enforcement agencies when Security requires assistance? Is there a list of situations in which Security might need such assistance? Is a decision-tree available for such contingencies? (See Chapter 2.)
- If Security personnel provide traffic control, are there procedures to follow when officers are needed elsewhere?

Section XI Internal Disaster

This section involves a number of subsections. The manual should contain prescriptive information for each.

1. Fire Procedures
2. Patient Evacuation Procedures
3. Physical Plant Damage Control

- power supply
- gas supply
- water supply

1. Fire Procedures

Every facility must fully develop and disseminate fire evacuation procedures and maps. General evacuation maps as well as unit evacuation maps should be included in the manual. They also should be replicated and posted in prominent places throughout the institution. Procedures should be stated clearly and in simple language. The easier an instruction is to follow, the more likely that losses can be minimized. The following excerpt from the procedure for an Accounting Department is illustrative:

> Type: *Fire Emergency*
> Code Red: Day, evening, night
> (1) Remain calm.
> (2) Close all windows.
> (3) Turn off all machines but *do not turn off lights.*
> (4) Remove "Fire Removal" labeled records.
> (5) Return all files to cabinets and lock.
> (6) Assemble in South Corridor until all-clear or other instruction is given.
> (7) Evacuate, using South Corridor or 7th Street stairs.

Fire procedures can be assembled in diagram, narrative, checklist, or any combination of formats. An excellent comprehensive fire safety procedure developed by a tertiary care hospital is reprinted in Appendix 4–E, Exhibit A. It details procedures, types of fires, and a fire drill procedure.

2. Patient Evacuation Procedures

Evacuation is a serious decision, fraught with risk. Evacuation means the movement either within the facility, or outside of it, from a dangerous or potentially dangerous area to a place of comparative safety. This subsection of the manual should define criteria for evacuation:

Partial Evacuation Mode. Patients at risk in their own room are moved to another room.

Lateral Evacuation Mode. This involves moving patients away from a fire or other threat in a nearby room or unit. Wheelchair, bed, blanket, and stretcher may be used. Ambulatory patients should be instructed to form a chain by holding hands and follow a staff member assigned to evacuate them. After evacuation, rooms and corridors should be checked for remaining patients and personnel. If the threat is fire, all doors, corridor cutoffs, and windows should be closed.

Downward Evacuation Mode. In this mode patients are moved downward, away from a threat in upper floors. Fire doors should be closed behind evacuees.

Facility Evacuation Mode. This involves the total evacuation of the facility. In most buildings, evacuation requires use of all stairways. Most communities have ordinances prohibiting elevator use during a fire. Evacuation should take place one floor at a time, with instruction by dedicated internal communication line or by messenger.

Evacuation routes from each unit should be depicted clearly in a map with accompanying instructions. Exhibit 4–21 is an example of evacuation instructions.

Some manuals give specific instructions for removal of patients. An excellent example of such procedures is reprinted from the manual of a major medical center (Appendix 4–E, Exhibit B).

Occasionally a facility has to discharge patients to make room for incoming disaster victims. The following are key questions to consider in developing this subsection of the manual.

- Is there a policy/procedure for the "early" discharge of admitted patients? Does the policy/procedure specify criteria for determining those who can be discharged?
- Who is authorized to approve transfer or discharge of inpatients if private physicians cannot be reached?
- Are there mutual transfer agreements with adjacent facilities? Has an agreement been developed with the local disaster communications agency for

---

Exhibit 4–21 Example of Evacuation Instruction for a Treatment Department

---

PEDIATRIC DEPARTMENT

1. *Person Responsible*
   a. Pediatric Nursing Coordinator
   b. or Unit Charge Nurse on duty
2. *Items to Be Hand-Carried during Evacuation:*
   a. Medical records
   b. Controlled drugs
3. *Priority Personnel Responsibilities:*
   a. Patient evacuation
   b. Removal of medical records and controlled drugs
4. *Evacuation Route*
   a. Primary Route—move toward the rear of the building along Blue Corridor, take 2nd Street stairwell to parking lot.
   b. Secondary Route—move to south side of building along Green Corridor, take 1st Street stairwell to street.

appropriate transfer in the event adjacent institutions cannot honor previously established agreements because of structural damage or overload?

- Are there procedures for expediting forms? Has a community transfer sheet been developed for continuity and familiarity?
- How will relatives be notified of patient relocation? Who will handle inquiries from relatives?
- Have alternate prior transportation arrangements been made (taxi, bus, van), since normal transportation modes may be inaccessible during a disaster?
- Has a traffic route been identified for transport vehicles dispatched for patient evacuation? (It should not conflict with incoming casualty rescue vehicles.)
- Have criteria been developed for transfer decisions for casualties after triage in the Triage Area?
- Does the manual(s) contain an appropriate list of referral facilities (i.e., burns) and their criteria for receipt? Have transfer agreements been reviewed by the local disaster communication center, if that agency provides casualty distribution coordination?
- Have procedures been developed to guide the transfer process? Are appropriate paper work and notification procedures available?
- What will the inhouse system be for communication of relocation, transfer, evacuation, and discharge activities to the Command Post, Public Information Center, and Admitting?
- Have contingency evacuation plans been developed in the event of destruction and hazard within the facility? For example, has an alternate route been established if an exit route fails because of structural damage to the facility?
- How will acutely ill patients be transferred if specialized equipment and/or personnel are required for safe transport?
- Where will inhouse patients be collected to await transport if they must be held outside the building because of structural damage, fire, or during a bomb investigation? Have special needs been anticipated?

3. Physical Plant Damage Control

The facility's Engineering Department plays an essential role in both internal and external disasters. This subsection of the manual must specify procedures and materials for:

- structural check and checklists
- securing doors, blocking off hazardous areas
- securing or relocating the Triage Area and Emergency Department in the event an internal radiation or hazardous chemical disaster in the facility itself makes them inoperable

- securing elevators
- securing power, gas, and water supplies
- obtaining stored equipment from facility storage areas.

If the institution does not have onsite engineering personnel, procedures must be developed that specify who will perform the initial facility check, how engineering personnel will be notified, and how hazardous- or security-important areas will be contained.

Section XII Community Interface

This section has four subsections:

1. Media Relations Center/Public Information Center
2. Public Safety
3. Ambulance
4. Red Cross and other agencies.

Procedures should be developed for each subsection.

1. Media Relations Center/Public Information Center

Whenever a disaster strikes, the news media become integrally involved. Facilities receiving casualties or cooperating in the response in any way should expect to receive media inquiries. Even when drills are held, the media generally are interested, particularly if the exercises involve community resources.

The most appropriate way to handle questions from the media is to refer all calls to the area designated by the facility plan as a Media Relations Center. Procedures should be developed that:

- designate a spokesperson for the facility
- identify radio/TV news broadcast times and newspaper publication times
- locate the Media Relations Center in a part of the facility where there is ample space for press briefings without interference in disaster operations
- prepare news releases using a format contained in the manual.

In preparing this subsection of the manual, the following questions should be considered.

- Who will respond to media inquiries?
- Has an appropriate site been established as a Media Relations Center? This site must not provide access to treatment areas, the Command Post, and the Triage Area.

- How will authorized media representatives be identified? Who will be responsible for checking credentials? When and where will credentials be checked?
- What format will be followed in releasing casualty information? Who will be authorized to release such information and to act as facility spokesperson?
- Where and when will press conferences be held? Who will be the authorized spokesperson? What information can be released?
- Is there a procedure for the release of statements in writing and/or over the telephone?
- Is there a policy for the use of photographic and camera equipment in the facility? How will consents from casualties be handled if media personnel photograph or film them?
- Have the media been instructed regarding appropriate entry and access to the facility? Is there a written policy/procedure for this activity that also dictates when and where media will not be allowed access?
- Does the plan identify parking facilities for media representatives? Does the parking area provide sufficient room for the large equipment vehicles (such as TV vans) that the media might use?

Facility personnel should cooperate with the media to every extent possible. Policy/procedures for doing so should be clearly specified and reviewed with the local media before a disaster event. Disruption of patient care and invasion of patients' rights must be avoided. While the Command Post can provide some information about the status of the intake of casualties and their treatment, it is the Media Relations Center that should act as the locus of information on the facility's response.

Some institutions establish a Public Information Center (PIC) to provide family members with information about victims. While the PIC also serves to provide vital information on the status of the intake of casualties and their treatment, it should be operated as an entity separate from the Media Relations Center. The distraught relative who comes to the PIC to inquire about a family member but is confronted by a newsperson instead can suffer extraordinary emotional pain. Victims and families must be shielded from inappropriate and intrusive behavior by the media as well as by others.

Providing public information to the public is subject to the same risks as providing it to the media. The numbers of visitors increase in times of disaster. Those with inpatient relatives not directly involved in the disaster want to verify that their family member is OK. Those with family members or friends who are casualties will come to determine their status. To avoid error in the information presented and to provide efficient generation of such information, the PIC should follow specific procedures. Relatives seeking information will need sympathetic and timely help as well as emotional support.

The PIC should be located close to the area where qualified counselors (social workers, clergy, and/or psychiatric clinicians) are stationed. However, the site should not be where people can wander into treatment areas. Restrooms and rest areas should be close by. The entire area must be securable.

Other issues this subsection of the manual should address are:

- Who will establish the PIC and at what point in time in relation to the disaster notification?
- What criteria will be used in deciding to open the PIC?
- Where will the PIC be located? Is there an alternate location in the event the primary one is unsafe?
- How will access by relatives/friends/concerned citizens be controlled? Which entry are they to use?
- Who will staff the PIC? Who will be authorized to act as a spokesperson for the facility?
- How will PIC personnel be identified? Will designated PIC personnel be separately identifiable to the public, since other staff members may be in and out of the area?
- Is there a communications link with the Command Post?
- Are there policies/procedures to govern release of information, expediting of patient status information, visitation to casualties and nondisaster inpatients during the event, overnight stays by relatives?
- Are there appropriate personnel for counselling of distraught relatives? Will the relatives be managed in the Center or elsewhere? Has that other area been identified?
- Is there a contingency plan for the PIC if the building's restrooms and/or plumbing are damaged?
- How will the food needs of relatives be handled? Are they to use the facility cafeteria? How will that affect food services that are attempting to meet increased demand from staff?
- Has a list of supplies that might be needed by relatives been determined? Are such items as blankets, medications, cots, telephone equipment, and bottled water available?

Section XIII Special Incidents

This subsection involves specific responses to incidents such as bomb threats, earthquakes, severe weather, terrorism, hazardous chemical/radiation accidents, and civil disorder. Specific procedures must be developed for each and included in the manual. Examples of three different sets of procedures (severe weather, bomb threat, earthquake), each prepared by a different health facility, are presented in Appendix 4–F, Exhibits A, B, C, and D. Note the differences in the formats.

Section XIV Attachments

Attachments are the documents, blank forms, sample forms, and diagrams that are referenced in the manual but are not directly a part of the text. The following are typical subsections:

1. Disaster Training Plan
2. Cost–Recovery Procedures
3. Long-Term Disaster Response
4. Managing the Stress of Disaster
5. Evacuation Maps/Instructions
6. Location of Shut-Off Valves

1. Disaster Training Plan

The manual should contain an annual training plan. (For a detailed discussion, see Chapter 5.)

2. Cost–Recovery Procedures

Disasters have a marked financial impact because they disrupt routines and necessitate extraordinary costs. If the facility itself is the victim of the event, the financial impact can vary, predicated on the amount of damage the structure receives, the numbers of patients discharged, the number of casualties treated, the numbers of personnel used and hours worked, the amount of supplies utilized, the amount of equipment malfunction or destruction in both the disaster and the haste of the response, and the ability to recoup lost revenues after the event.

Some reimbursement may be available from federal sources if a general disaster is declared (and the facility is damaged) and/or from insurance companies. But such reimbursement rarely matches costs. Some patient care costs can be recovered from third parties such as Blue Cross, Medicare, and other insurance carriers; however, in a disaster, patients must be treated first and then, once stabilized, they undergo the usual financial eligibility admitting screening procedure.

The institution must anticipate costs and plan to minimize losses. In preparing this subsection of the manual there are several questions to consider:

- Does the plan, in an effort to minimize loss and damage to equipment, address specifically what to do with malfunctioning equipment, how to recognize loss of its integrity and request replacement before damage is irreversible, and the method to follow when equipment is lent from one area to another?

- What, if any, arrangements have been considered or established by adjacent facilities to minimize their loss of revenue during a disaster or to recoup costs?
- What criteria have been established by local, regional, state, and federal sources for facility reimbursement? Will procedures have to be developed to ensure that the institution documents, both progressively and retrospectively, areas in which it meets criteria?
- Have procedures been developed, and mutual aid agreements established, for lending or borrowing supplies and equipment between and among facilities?
- How and when will vending companies be reimbursed for deliveries required during the event. Are agreements in writing?
- Who will be responsible for equipment/supply inventories and documentation of utilization?
- How will charges for disaster casualty care be tracked in the facility?
- How will staff time be managed, tracked, and paid?
- How will the cost of services for relatives and nonpatients be determined and recovered?
- What losses will be considered acceptable and reasonable by the controller?
- Will costs of rescue vehicle resupply be charged? If so, to whom?

3. Long-Term Disaster Response

Large-scale disasters that affect the community and/or region will result in long-term consequences that have implications for:

- sanitation
- infectious disease control
- shelter requirements for staff, relatives, delayed category victims
- food and water depletion/supply and equipment depletion
- longer period of facility overload before state/federal aid is available
- psychological sequels for staff, victims, and relatives.

The American Red Cross and Civil Defense authorities are integral factors in survivor relocation and emergency sanitation. However, the facility may be in a "self-help" situation for days or weeks before these agencies and/or the military can be of major assistance to all affected areas and citizens. Because health care facilities represent help, uninjured community survivors also may come in seeking food and shelter. While admittedly a disaster of this magnitude is less likely to occur, the plan and manual must address such a possibility. The following questions may help identify areas for this subsection of the manual.

- Have additional resources for food and water been identified in the event of a long-term disaster? Can the facility provide, without outside help, at least 30 days of sufficient food, water, pharmaceuticals, and patient care supplies for casualties, inpatients, staff, and relatives? Have priorities been established for who will receive supplies if they become limited without possibility of reinforcement for hours or days?
- Has a procedure been established for the purification of existing water (i.e., from toilets, freezers)?
- Are enough clean, closed, noncorrodible containers available for storage of purified water?
- Have procedures been developed to identify diminished water resources and prevent utilization of existing supplies for hygiene use? (See Exhibit 4–22.)
- Has a contingency plan been developed to meet the need for sleep areas and clothing for staff and stranded relatives? Where will civilians be placed if they arrive in need of shelter only? How will food, water, and clothing be distributed to these survivors?
- Who will manage infectious disease control in the disaster aftermath? What procedures will be enforced to prevent development and spread of disease?
- How will sanitation practices be conducted if all available water must be retained for drinking? Are there alternative washup supplies such as foam products and packaged Handi Wipes?
- How will psychological needs of patients, relatives, and staff be met?
- How will the bodies be handled if staff members have been killed while on duty? How will they be handled if they are injured? Who will replace them in patient care? How will the psychological needs of co-workers be managed?
- How will staff members distraught over the whereabouts or condition of family members and friends be dealt with?

4. Managing the Stress of Disaster

Stress is an endemic problem in any disaster. Even the most experienced health professional can be affected adversely. In anticipation, some facilities specify activities to be undertaken in the postdisaster period:

- "debriefing" discussion groups
- referring personnel for psychological help
- anticipating the possibility that victims received may be friends and relatives of personnel on duty and formulating plans to handle such situations

Exhibit 4–22 Example of Procedures for Managing Disruption of the Water
Supply

Water Delivery

1. If the disruption exceeds six hours, arrangement has been made with (insert name and telephone number of water vendor) to provide a tank truck.
2. Water supplied in the tank truck will be used to keep the boilers operating and supplying steam.
   a. The volume in the holding tank that feeds the boilers will last 8 to 12 hours after disruption of service.
   b. The hospital has sufficient equipment to pump the water from the tank truck to the holding tank.

Water Distribution and Delivery

1. Upon disruption, the Engineering Department will coordinate distribution of bottled water in five-gallon containers from inventory as follows:

	Number of Bottles
a. Central Service	3
b. Dietary	5
c. Laboratory	3
d. Pharmacy	2
e. Radiology	1
f. Respiratory Services	2
g. Special Care Unit	5
h. Nursing Units (2)	5/unit

2. The hospital has made arrangements with _____ _____, to provide a full truck of bottled water (144 five-gallon bottles) within 6 hours of notification. The hospital would be given priority as additional requirements were determined.
3. The engineer on duty will instruct all departments to alter their operations as much as possible to minimize the use of water, as follows:
   a. Dietary would go to all-disposable dishes and utensils to eliminate the need to operate the dishwasher.
   b. Nursing would go to P.M. care on all shifts, eliminating baths.

- developing criteria for determining desirable work-rest periods during an event.

Current literature suggests that rescue workers invariably continue to work even when they have sustained severe personal losses in a disaster. However, the resulting psychological conflict makes them extremely vulnerable to stress reactions. These may be manifested as severe fatigue, hostility, hysteria, crying, confusion, denial, and withdrawal, as well as somatic problems. Both acute and delayed psychological reactions may produce "aftershocks" for a long time. Morale and the "rescue spirit" may be reduced significantly. Because coping skills vary widely among individuals, access to a trained and experienced mental health specialist is vital to the adequate performance of stressed staff members.

It should be noted, too, that mental health professionals are not immune to adverse reactions to disaster. The same is true for ED personnel.

Emergency Department personnel, faced with receipt of injured or dead rescue workers with whom they may have had an intimate working relationship, are prime candidates for acute stress reactions. In small communities, ED personnel may also have to manage dead or injured friends and relatives as well. There are no easy answers to the dilemma of severe psychological stress in disaster response. Psychological debriefings are invaluable in the management of shock and denial and as a means of diffusing anger. Grief, guilt, and confusion may be delayed for days or weeks but can be diminished in intensity by immediate crisis intervention and emotional ventilation and support. Those involved will need to know that the variety of physical, cognitive, and emotional symptoms they are experiencing is normal to survivors of any disaster. (See Chapter 6 for further discussion of stress and appropriate interventions.)

SUMMARY

This chapter has provided a format and guidelines for developing a model disaster manual. No single format will work for every institution. A comprehensive manual replete with examples and diagrams may be workable for some organizations and unworkable for others. The intent here is to suggest and present major sections and subsections, including examples and samples. Additional references are in the Appendixes to this chapter.

The following are tips about the manual and its format

1. Keep It Simple

New and veteran staff members and other employees will not have the time to read lengthy procedures in a manual during an actual event. The manner in which the manual is written is critical to efficient response. The "ideal" disaster manual is easily identified by a distinctive cover and its contents should be arranged so that information can be obtained rapidly.

A loose-leaf binding will simplify revisions. All pages (and updates) should be dated and numbered. A record of any changes should be kept—a good place for it is in a cover sleeve.

While a health facility disaster manual may have sections referring to specific departments or patient-care units, each department or unit should have its own separately bound minimanual. The minimanual should be easily accessible at the work site to maximize start-up responses.

The minimanual for each department, at a minimum, should specify:

- unit responsibility during a disaster
- chain of command
- callback procedure and documentation
- assignment procedure and sample assignment sheet
- disaster action cards
- patient evacuation procedures and routes
- procedures for receipt and management of casualties
- procedures for request/procurement/repair/transfer of supplies/equipment
- interface with facility and community resources.

2. Use a Consistent Format

Even though staff members may have to refer to the unit manual during an event to answer operational questions, they should be so thoroughly trained in the concept of disaster response that referral to the overall institutional manual is minimal. If that manual is used, however, its material should be easy to find, read, and comprehend. Tabs for quick reference should be used to identify specific areas so it will not be necessary to refer to the inside table of contents or summary. Definitions for technical terms should be included if they are not everyday words, such as "triage," "moulage" (using make-up and molds to depict injuries), "casualty," etc., or if they refer to activities that are not ordinary procedures. Color coding of information is a dramatic way to define specific areas of the manual but will not be particularly helpful unless personnel have been exposed already to the manual and its utilization before they search for information.

3. Use General Headings

Although patient care areas and support services should have the general manual in their departments at all times, individual departments and unit sections should be designated separately. A copy of the manual must be available to the staff 24 hours a day, not tucked into a supervisor's office or on the desk of the Disaster Planning Coordinator. Even if it is being revised, the actual working manual should remain in the unit.

4. Keep Command Chains and Notification Lists Simple

Personnel should be designated by title rather than by name because individuals frequently are reassigned or leave (and are replaced by new persons) but disaster plans usually are not updated as often. To simplify use of the manual, callback sheets that contain current personnel rosters should be maintained in a standard location in the department or unit. The callback sheet should be revised each time there are personnel changes.

Some facilities include the callback sheet in their unit disaster manuals and on a clipboard stored with the unit's disaster supplies. Although command chains and callback lists might well be found in the manual, they also should be available outside it on such a clipboard so that staff members do not have to search through the book for them. Unit plans should reflect only notification lists pertinent to them. Color-coding departmental callback lists to indicate residential distances— 5, 15, and 30 minutes from the institution—and structuring the work sheet by shifts will facilitate calling appropriate individuals to obtain help quickly. The callback work sheet should be separated from the manual so that those assigned to call do not have to search the manual for it.

5. Disaster Action Cards

The manual should specify roles and responsibilities. A convenient way to do so is to detail them on Disaster Action Cards. The cards should be stored separately from the manual for ease in distribution and use.

NOTES

1. Emily Friedman, "Updating Disaster Plans: A Tale of Three Hospitals," *Hospitals* 52 (May 1978): 95.

2. Joint Commission on Accreditation of Hospitals, *Accreditation Manual for Hospitals, 1985.* (Chicago: Author, 1984), 132–133.

3. Jeffrey R. MacDonald, MD. Principles of Field Triage. Lecture at St. Mary's Hospital, Long Beach, CA, 1978.

JCAH Disaster Planning Requirements for Hospitals

Standard V

The hospital has an emergency preparedness program designed to provide for the effective utilization of available resources so that patient care can be continued during a disaster.

Required Characteristics

A. A hospital designated as a disaster emergency center by a local authority such as the fire department or Civil Defense agency has an emergency preparedness program that addresses disasters both external and internal to the hospital.   20

B. Concise, preestablished, documented plans to be implemented during a disaster are established through the emergency preparedness program.

   1. Emergency preparedness plans provide for the effective utilization   25
   of available resources to prevent or minimize the consequences of a disaster.

   2. Emergency preparedness plans are pertinent to a variety of disasters and are based on the hospital's capabilities and limitations.

C. The role of the hospital in communitywide disaster plans is identified in   30
   the emergency preparedness program.

D. The emergency preparedness program addresses hospital preparedness, including space utilization, supplies, communication systems, security, and utilities.

Source: Reprinted from *Accreditation Manual for Hospitals, 1985*, pp. 132–133, with permission of the Joint Commission on Accreditation of Hospitals, © 1985.

E. The emergency preparedness program addresses staff preparedness, including staffing requirements and the designation of roles and functions, particularly in terms of capabilities and limitations.

F. All hospital personnel are provided with appropriate training.

G. The emergency preparedness program addresses patient management, including modified schedules, criteria for the cessation of nonessential services, and patient transfer determinations, particularly in terms of discharge and relocation.   5

H. The emergency preparedness program is implemented, evaluated, and documented semiannually.   10

   1. Each implementation (whether a drill or an actual emergency) exercises emergency preparedness plan elements related to hospital preparedness, staff preparedness, and patient management; at least one implementation includes an influx of patients from outside the hospital.

   2. Documentation includes, at the least, problems identified during implementation, corrective actions taken, and staff participation.   15

I. There is a fire plan that addresses the use and function of fire alarm and detection systems, containment, and the protection of lives, including movement transfer to areas of refuge, evacuation plans, and fire extinguishment. It is recommended that on each work shift the hospital have appropriately trained personnel responsible for assisting with the   20 implementation of the fire plan and the activation of the nonautomatic components of the fire safety systems.

J. The fire plan is implemented at least quarterly for each work shift of hospital personnel in each patient-occupied building.   25

   1. Documentation of the implementation of the plan includes, at a minimum, problems identified during implementation, corrective actions taken, and staff participation.

K. Hospital employees and staff are provided with appropriate education and training in elements of the emergency preparedness program and in   30 elements of the fire plan.

L. The emergency preparedness program is evaluated annually and is updated as needed.

Appendix 4–B

SNF Disaster Plan Standards in California

72551. External Disaster and Mass Casualty Program.*

(a) A written external disaster and mass casualty program plan shall be adopted and followed. The plan shall be developed with the advice and assistance of county or regional and local planning offices and shall not conflict with county and community disaster plan. A copy of the plan shall be available on the premises for review by the Department [the California Department of Health Services].

(b) The plan shall provide procedures in event of community and widespread disasters. The written plan shall include at least the following:

(1) Sources of emergency utilities and supplies, including gas, water, food, and essential medical supportive materials.

(2) Procedures for assigning personnel and recalling off-duty personnel.

(3) Unified medical command. A chart of lines of authority in the facility.

(4) Procedures for the conversion of all usable space into areas for patient observation and immediate care of emergency admissions.

(5) Prompt transfer of casualties when necessary and after preliminary medical or surgical services have been rendered, to the facility most appropriate for administering definitive care. Procedures for moving patients from damaged areas of the facility to undamaged areas.

(6) Arrangements for provision of transportation of patients including emergency housing where indicated. Procedures for emergency transfers of patients who can be moved to other health facilities, including arrangements for safe and efficient transportation and transfer information.

(7) Procedures for emergency discharge of patients who can be discharged without jeopardy into the community, including prior arrangements for their care,

---

*Title 22, California Administrative Code, 1985.

125

arrangements for safe and efficient transportation and at least one follow-up inquiry within 24 hours to ascertain that patients are receiving required care.

(8) Procedures for maintaining a record of patient relocation.

(9) An evacuation plan, including evacuation routes, emergency phone numbers of physicians, health facilities, the fire department and local emergency medical services agencies, and arrangements for the safe transfer of patients after evacuation.

(10) A tag containing all pertinent personal and medical information which shall accompany each patient who is moved, transferred, discharged or evacuated.

(11) Procedures for maintaining security in order to keep relatives, visitors, and curious persons out of the facility during a disaster.

(12) Procedures for providing emergency care to incoming patients from other health facilities.

(13) Assignment of public relations liaison duties to a responsible individual employed by the facility to release information to the public during a disaster.

(c) The plan shall be reviewed at least annually and revised as necessary to ensure that the plan is current. All personnel shall be instructed in the requirements of the plan. There shall be evidence in the personnel files or the orientation checklist indicating that all new employees have been oriented to the plan and procedures at the beginning of their employment.

(d) The facility shall participate in all local and state disaster drills and test exercises when asked to do so by the local or state disaster or emergency medical services agencies.

(e) A disaster drill shall be held by the facility at six-month intervals. There shall be a written report of the facility's participation in each drill or test exercise. Staff from all shifts shall participate in drills or test exercises.

NOTE: Authority cited: Sections 208(a) and 1275, Health and Safety Code. Reference Section 1276, Health and Safety Code.

*   *   *   *   *

72553. Fire and Internal Disasters.

(a) A written fire and internal disaster plan incorporating evacuation procedures shall be developed with the assistance of qualified fire, safety and other appropriate experts. A copy of the plan shall be available on the premises for review by the staff and the Department.

(b) The written plan shall include at least the following:

(1) Procedures for the assignment of personnel to specific tasks and responsibilities.

(2) Procedures for the use of alarm systems and signals.

(3) Procedures for fire containment.

(4) Priority for notification of staff, including names and telephone numbers.

(5) Location of firefighting equipment.

(6) Procedures for evacuation and specification of evacuation routes.

(7) Procedures for moving patients from damaged areas of the facility to undamaged areas.

(8) Procedures for emergency transfer of patients who can be moved to other health facilities, including arrangements for safe and efficient transportation.

(9) Procedures for emergency discharge of patients who can be discharged without jeopardy into the community, including prior arrangements for their care, arrangements for safe and efficient transportation and at least one follow-up inquiry within 24 hours to ascertain that patients are receiving their required care.

(10) A disaster tag containing all pertinent personal and medical information to accompany each patient who is moved, transferred, discharged or evacuated.

(11) Procedures for maintaining a record of patient relocation.

(12) Procedures for handling incoming or relocated patients.

(13) Other provisions as dictated by circumstances.

(c) Fire and internal disaster drills shall be held at least quarterly, under varied conditions for each individual shift of the facility personnel. The actual evacuation of patients to safe areas during a drill is optional.

(d) The evacuation plan shall be posted throughout the facility and shall include at least the following:

(1) Evacuation routes.

(2) Location of fire alarm boxes.

(3) Location of fire extinguishers.

(4) Emergency telephone number of the local fire department.

(e) A dated, written report and evaluation of each drill and rehearsal shall be maintained and shall include signatures of all employees who participated.

*   *   *   *   *

72641. Emergency Lighting and Power System.

(a) Auxiliary lighting and power facilities shall be provided as required by Sections E702-5, E702-6, E702-8 and E702-21 of Title 24, California Administrative Code. Flashlights shall be in readiness for use at all times. Open-flame type of light shall not be used.

(b) The licensee shall provide and maintain an emergency electrical system in safe operating condition and in compliance with subsections (d), (e), and (f). The system shall serve all lighting, signals, alarms, and equipment required to permit continued operation of all necessary functions of the facility for a minimum of six hours.

(c) If the Department determined that an evaluation of the emergency electrical system of a facility or portion thereof is necessary, the Department may require the licensee to submit a report by a registered electrical engineer which shall establish a basis for alteration of the system to provide reasonable compliance with Subarticle E702-B, Part 3, Title 24, California Administrative Code (Emergency Electrical Systems for Existing Nursing Homes). Essential engineering data, including load calculations, assumptions and tests, and where necessary, plans and specifications, acceptable to the Department, shall be submitted in substantiation of the report. When corrective action is determined to be necessary, the work shall be initiated and completed within an acceptable time limit.

(d) The emergency lighting and power system shall be maintained in operating condition to provide automatic restoration of power for emergency circuits within ten seconds after normal power failure.

(e) Emergency generators shall be tested at least every 14 days under full load condition for a minimum of 30 minutes.

(f) A written record of inspection, performance, exercising period and repair of the emergency electrical system shall be regularly maintained on the premises and available for inspection by the Department.

Appendix 4–C

Exhibit A: Sample Disaster Tag

ATTACH SECURELY TO PATIENT

Pink copy: administration	
White copy: admitting	
Hard copy: patient record	NO. 524873

Hospital: *St. Josephina*

Patient name (Last)	(First)	(Middle)
Smith	*Donald*	*K.*

Address

1252 N. 11th St.

Date	Time	Age	Sex	Religion
10/5/86	*1015*	*32*	*M*	*Cath.*

Description of patient: (Ht, Wt, Eyes, Hair, Compl, Marks, Clothing)

6 ft. brn./green 180# Cauc
torn blue shirt, brn. trousers. blk shoes/socks

ALLERGIES:
Horse Serum

Next of kin:
(name)   (address)

Alice Smith   *1252 N 11th St.*   *Wife*

129

Exhibit A continued

INITIAL ASSESSMENT:

2° burns face/hands
Open Chest Wound Ⓡ Chest
Rigid belly, responds purposefully to voice

INITIAL TREATMENT:

☐ Airway   ☑ IV *RK 1000 cc*
☑ Bleeding control   ☑ Oxygen *@ 9L/min mask*
☐ Tourniquet   ☐ Medication:
☐ Splint
☑ OTHER: *vaseline gauge dressing, occlusive*
                                        bandage

INITIAL ROUTING AT HOSPITAL TRIAGE POINT:

☑ Surgery   ☐ Emergency Department   ☐ Observation area
☐ X-ray   ☐ ICU   ☐ Morgue
☐ First aid   ☐ CCU   OTHER:

PRIORITY DESIGNATION

☑ Immediate   If immediate care affix
☐ Delayed   RED   RED LABEL
☐ Dead   If delayed care affix
                                         BLACK LABEL

DO NOT DETACH TAG FROM PATIENT UNTIL INCORPORATED IN PATIENT
RECORD
SEE REVERSE SIDE FOR TREATMENT, DISPOSITION, AND INSTRUCTIONS

Source: Reprinted from "Disaster Management" by J.K. Simoneau in *Emergency Nursing: Principles and Practice,* 2nd ed., S.A. Sheehy and J.M. Barber (Eds.), with permission of the C.V. Mosby Company, St. Louis, © 1985.

Appendix 4–C

Exhibit B: Sample Triage Casualty Log

Time to Triage	Tag No.	Name	Priority	Initial Disposition	Time Out	Final Disposition	Diagnosis

Source: Reprinted from "Disaster Management" by J.K. Simoneau in *Emergency Nursing: Principles and Practice*, 2nd ed., S.A. Sheehy and J.M. Barber (Eds.), with permission of the C.V. Mosby Company, St. Louis, © 1985.

Appendix 4–C

Exhibit C: Sample Disaster Casualty Disposition Log

PATIENT NAME	LOCATION	TIME OUT	DISPOSITION	TIME RECEIVED
1.				
2.				
3.				
4.				
5.				
6.				
7.				
8.				
9.				
10.				
11.				
12.				
13.				
14.				
15.				
16.				
17.				
18.				
19.				
20.				
21.				
22.				
23.				
24.				
25.				

Appendix 4–C

Exhibit D: Hourly Individual Area Disaster Status

COMPLETE AND FORWARD COPY TO COMMAND POST EVERY HOUR

Time _____ Date _____ Person completing _____

Department _____

Total beds now: _____ Total # of patients now: _____

Total nursing staff now: _____ physicians present now _____

    Transporters/messengers _____ clerks _____

Name of supervising person now directing the area: _____

Equipment needs:

Supply needs:

Personnel needs:

Evacuation activity:

Patient name/#	Where sent	How	Time

COMMENTS:

Appendix 4–C

Exhibit E: Sample Implementation Status Form

To Be Completed by Administrator Mobilizing Facility

Date _____ Time _____ Notified by: _____

Administrator: _____

Initial Code Announcement: GREEN   YELLOW   RED

Time announcement made _____

Code change: YES/NO   Time _____ Code _____

Beds available: Total now _____ 15 minutes _____ 30 minutes _____

          60 minutes _____ 2 hours _____ 4 hours _____

Specialty beds available NOW:

    ICU _____ Recovery room _____ Surgical suites _____

    CCU _____ Emergency Department _____

Areas mobilized/Time:

    Triage _____ Command Post _____ ED Command Post _____ ED _____

    Urgent care _____ Delayed care _____ Surgery _____ X-ray _____

    Lab _____ Personnel Pool _____ Security _____ Press/media _____

Engineering facility check time begun _____ finished _____

    Comments:

Amount of blood on hand _____ Resource contacted/time: _____

Time evacuation begun: _____

    From _____ To _____ Time _____ # _____

    From _____ To _____ Time _____ # _____

    From _____ To _____ Time _____ # _____

COMMENTS:

White copy: Command Post/Administration. Pink: Retain as work sheet.

Appendix 4–C

Exhibit F: Sample Personnel Check-In and Assignment Roster

Name	Category	Area/Duty	Changes	Reporting Time On Duty	Off Duty
Cathy J.	RN	Treatment area Disaster coordinator		already here	
Clark S.	MD	Treatment area Disaster officer		1010	
Jack L.	MD	Triage physician		1015	
Lynn M.	RN	Treatment area Team 1		1012	
Tracy R.	RN	Triage nurse		1005	
Roger L.	ECT	Treatment area Team 1		1020	
Gary R.	ECT	Clinic	Treatment area	1020	
Nancy M.	RN	Clinic	Team 3 1040	1030	

Source: Reprinted from "Disaster Aspects of Emergency Nursing" by J.K. Simoneau in *Emergency Nursing: Principles and Practice*, 2nd ed., S.A. Sheehy and J.M. Barber (Eds.), with permission of C.V. Mosby Company, St. Louis, © 1985.

Appendix 4–C

Exhibit G: Sample Disaster Control Form

Request for Personnel/Supplies/Equipment

Type of Assistance	Area Requesting: Person Requesting: Request for:		Date: Time: Title:
	= Personnel	= Supplies	= Equipment
Personnel	Personnel type: Priority (circle one) 1 2 3 Comments:		# Needed:
Supplies	Supply type: Priority (circle one) 1 2 3 Comments:		Amount:
Equipment	Equipment type: Priority (circle one) 1 2 3 Comments:		

Priority 1 = Stat   Priority 2 = Urgent 1-4 hours   Priority 3 = Within Reasonable Time

White Copy: Administration Command Post.   Yellow Copy: Controller.
Pink Copy: Area Requesting.

136

Appendix 4–C

Exhibit H: Sample Disaster Action Cards: Triage Area

Triage Area Coordinator

You are responsible for the function and process of the Triage Area.
1. Liaison with the Command Post, maintaining close communication regarding the operation of triage.
2. Supervise the Triage Area workers.
3. Ensure adequate personnel, obtaining from Personnel Pool when necessary.
4. Ensure proper break times and appropriate scheduling.
5. Handle administrative problems such as equipment needs, coordinating with the Command Post all problem solutions which cannot be accomplished right in the area by the Coordinator.
6. Ensure proper maintenance of triage logs and statistics.
7. Ensure proper conduct of all triage procedures.
8. Coordinate patient flow with receiving areas.

Triage Officer

1. Evaluate each arriving casualty, performing a cursory primary survey (ABCs) and head-to-toe physical evaluation. Keep it brief, injury oriented, and focused on defining the problems and priorities.
2. Assign a triage category (Emergency, Urgent, Nonurgent).
3. Assign a triage disposition for further care.
4. DO NOT PERFORM TREATMENT EXCEPT FOR THE MOST ESSENTIAL LIFE-SAVING MANEUVERS.
5. DO NOT LEAVE YOUR AREA UNLESS RELIEVED BY ANOTHER TRIAGE OFFICER.
6. Wear your triage identification bib at all times.

Registered Nurse, Triage Area

1. Assist the Triage Officer in evaluation of casualties, including performance of a cursory physical exam.

137

Exhibit H continued

2. Assign triage categories in all cases you are evaluating by yourself (Emergent, Urgent, Nonurgent), and advise the Triage Officer of the category assigned.
3. Assign a triage disposition if necessary, log it in via the clerk, and advise the Triage Officer of your disposition.
4. Ensure that transport occurs immediately; assign a transporter if necessary.
5. Coordinate the ancillary workers on your team to complete their tasks efficiently and correctly.
6. Advise the Triage Coordinator of all equipment and supply needs at your station.
7. Wear your triage identification bib at all times.
8. DO NOT LEAVE YOUR AREA UNLESS RELIEVED BY THE TRIAGE COORDINATOR.

LVN, EMT-P, EMT-A

1. Assist the R.N. and Triage Officer in evaluating each casualty.
2. Obtain proper exam equipment and supplies as needed from the cart or shelves; advise the R.N. when supplies are running short.
3. Assist in disrobing and gowning casualties, and in obtaining clothing and valuables lists if the clerk needs assistance.
4. Apply oxygen as ordered by the R.N. or Triage Officer.
5. Wear your triage identification bib at all times.
6. DO NOT LEAVE THE TRIAGE STATION UNLESS RELIEVED BY THE TRIAGE COORDINATOR.

Clerk

1. Log each casualty into the Triage Log; ensure that all information required is complete unless that information is not currently available.
2. Dispatch messages as requested, utilizing the transporters or requesting a message runner from the Personnel Pool if the transporters are busy.
3. Obtain clothing and valuables lists as necessary; do not hold the casualty up to do so, however.
4. Bag clothing and valuables and ensure that they accompany the casualty to his disposition.
5. Wear your Triage identification bib at all times.
6. DO NOT LEAVE THE TRIAGE STATION UNLESS RELIEVED BY THE TRIAGE COORDINATOR.

Transporter

1. Transport casualties rapidly and safely from triage to their treatment disposition.
2. Wear your Triage identification bib at all times.
3. Return to your Triage station as soon as the patient is delivered to his/her disposition.
4. Advise the Triage Coordinator of all broken transport equipment.

Source: Reprinted from "Disaster Management" by J.K. Simoneau in *Emergency Nursing: Principles and Practice,* 2nd ed., S.A. Sheehy and J.M. Barber (Eds.), with permission of the C.V. Mosby Company, St. Louis, © 1985.

Appendix 4–D

Example of Triage Categories

TRIAGE CATEGORIES

In civilian triage, the maxim "sickest first" is used unless the Chief of Triage issues an order to use military triage terminology.

The following categories will be used:

Delayed

minor injuries such as small lacerations, single extremity injuries, foreign bodies imbedded in the skin of extremities unless near major vasculature, abrasions, minor burns (less than 5 percent third degree, or less than 20 percent second degree, or less than 30 percent first degree if none of these involve the airway, hands, feet, or genitalia).

Life Threatening

airway obstruction, shock with hemodynamic compromise, pulmonary or myocardial injury, massive hemorrhage, cardiac arrest in the triage area.

Emergent

open abdominal trauma, blunt abdominal trauma with hemodynamic compromise, head trauma with deterioration in level of consciousness, vascular compromise, second stage labor, major burns (over 5 percent third degree, over 20 percent second degree, over 30 percent first degree and any burns involving the airway, hands, feet, genitalia).

139

Urgent

fractures and dislocations that are open or that involve the hip or knee or are in association with other system injuries where the other injuries do not categorize into the EMERGENT category; eye injuries with impairment of vision; lacerations requiring debridement and repair of an extensive nature or that overlie a bony injury; facial injuries without airway interference.

Remember:

THE PRIMARY FUNCTION OF TRIAGE IS TO RAPIDLY ASSESS AND ASSIGN TREATMENT PRIORITIES AND DISPOSITION FOR TREATMENT.

TRIAGE IS A SERIAL PROCESS AND CATEGORIES FROM THE FIELD MAY HAVE TO BE CHANGED WHEN THE CASUALTY ARRIVES AT THE TRIAGE AREA.

PATIENTS MAY CHANGE CATEGORIES, DEPENDING ON THE DYNAMICS OF THEIR INJURIES AND THEIR RESPONSE TO THOSE INJURIES.

EVERYONE IN TRIAGE MUST BE AWARE OF THE CATEGORIES BEING USED AND WHAT INJURIES OR ILLNESSES FALL INTO THESE CATEGORIES.

Exhibit A: Saint Joseph Medical Center Fire Safety Procedure

INTRODUCTION

The rules and information in this fire safety protocol are to be put into effect immediately in the event a fire occurs at Saint Joseph Medical Center. All employees should know these general rules and also those specific instructions which apply to their position and assigned department. All must act as a team as the lives of patients and fellow employees may depend on effective actions. Above all "KEEP CALM." Act quickly, and quietly offer assurance to patients as may be necessary. Do not forget that fear and panic can do as much damage as the fire itself.

DIRECTIVES TO DEPARTMENT HEADS

A. Check periodically that:

1. Every member on your staff has read the fire manual and is oriented to his or her part in the plan.
2. All know how to give the fire alarm.
3. All know the location of the fire extinguishers and how to use them, and which kind to use for certain fires. Make arrangements with Plant Operations or Personnel Department regarding any staff members who have not been instructed in this.
4. All have knowledge of exits and which can be used for evacuation. Do NOT use the elevator.
5. All nursing service personnel are familiar with procedure on patient evacuation and that they know the "basic carries."
6. An alternate can take over in your absence.

GENERAL INFORMATION

A. Procedure of Reporting and Combating a Fire

1. Pull one fire alarm nearest to fire.
2. Call PBX by dialing *15* and give the operator your name, location of fire, type of fire, and its severity.

Source: Reprinted with permission from the *Disaster Manual* of St. Joseph Medical Center, Burbank, Cal.

Exhibit B: Emergency Removal of Patients

POLICY

Santa Monica Hospital Medical Center	POLICY NUMBER	6.7
	FUNCTIONAL AREA	Safety & Disaster Hospital Wide
	PAGE	1 OF 5

SUBJECT:	EFFECTIVE DATE	Form: 5/78 Rev: 10:80
EMERGENCY REMOVAL OF PATIENTS		
	APPROVED	

Under emergency conditions, the speed in which the patients must be removed from the building may be of paramount importance. To evacuate a building in a hurry will mean using all methods available to fit the situation. Manual carries will be included among these methods.

Through training and drilling, it has been proved that nurses can handle any of the removals or carries described. It takes some practice.

The method or carry used in any particular situation will vary with the conditions surrounding the emergency. Things to consider are:

1. Condition of patient
2. Nature of the emergency
3. Weight and size of patient (or nurse)
4. Height of bed
5. Number of patients to be relocated
6. Number of staff members available

Manual Carries

One Nurse

1. Blanket Carry
   a. Fold blanket diagonally.
   b. Pass folded blanket in back of patient; bring ends under arm. Tie blanket with square knot in front of patient, leaving enough slack to insert nurse's arm.
   c. Insert right arm, in upward movement, between knotted blanket and patient's chest.
   d. Turn back to patient, bend knees, and adjust blanket comfortably over right shoulder.

Exhibit B continued

POLICY

Santa Monica Hospital Medical Center

POLICY NUMBER	6.7
FUNCTIONAL AREA	Safety & Disaster Hospital Wide
PAGE	2 OF 5

SUBJECT:	EFFECTIVE Form: 5/78 Rev: 10/80
EMERGENCY REMOVAL OF PATIENTS	DATE
	APPROVED

    e. Straighten knees in order to lift patient from bed with minimum amount of strain or effort.

    f. Carry to safety.

2. Blanket Drag

    a. Unfold blanket.

    b. Place patient face up, diagonally on blanket.

    c. If patient is wearing shoes, remove them. This eliminates the possibility of heels catching on stairs and floor obstructions.

    d. Lift corner of blanket nearest to patient's head.

    e. Utilizing one or both hands, drag patient, head first, to place of safety. Patient evacuation down stairways can be accomplished rapidly by this method.

3. Pack Strap Method

Pull patient to sitting position, then grasp patient's right wrist with your left hand and patient's left wrist with your right hand. Duck your head under patient's arms without releasing wrists. Place your back against patient's chest so that your shoulders are lower than other's armpits. Then pull patient's arms over your shoulders and across your chest for leverage. Keep patient's wrists firmly grasped with either one or both hands. Lean forward slightly, straighten your knees, and transport patient to safety.

4. Hip Method

Sit on bed; turn patient on side facing you; place your back against patient's abdomen; grasp knees with one arm and slide your other arm down and across patient's back under free arm, grip patient under armpit; straighten your knees; draw patient up on hip; and carry to safety.

5. Cradle Drop (to blanket)

Unfold blanket on floor; face bed; lower your body with one knee up and one knee on floor—uppermost knee should be at right angles to patient's knees, rigid, and touching bed; grasp patient's knees with one arm and neck and shoulders with the other; do NOT attempt to lift patient, simply pull toward you and ease patient toward the floor. Your raised knee will support patient's knees and legs and your arm will support the shoulders and head. The cradle formed by your arm and knee will protect patient's back. Ease patient to blanket.

Exhibit B continued

POLICY

Santa Monica
Hospital
Medical Center

POLICY NUMBER	6.7
FUNCTIONAL AREA	Safety & Disaster Hospital Wide
PAGE	3 OF 5

SUBJECT:	EFFECTIVE DATE	Form: 5/78 Rev: 10/80
EMERGENCY REMOVAL OF PATIENTS	APPROVED	

6. Kneel Drop (to blanket)

   Unfold blanket on floor; face bed; lower body on both knees in kneeling position; grasp patient's knees with one arm, head and shoulders with the other; do NOT lift; pull patient straight out from bed until body contacts your chest; allow patient to slide down your body to the cushion formed by your knees; ease to blanket and remove from room.

Two Nurses

7. Utilize Blanket Drag (2)

8. Extremity Method

   First nurse works hands and arms from behind patient under patient's armpits, then grips own wrists across patient's chest; second nurse pulls patient's ankles out from bed, then backs up between patient's knees and grasps both knees under own arms. Lift patient, and remove to safety.

9. Swing Method

   Pull patient to sitting position at right angles to bed with nurse on each side; both nurses pass one arm under patient's arm and across the back and secure a firm grip on each other's shoulders; the other arm is then passed under patient's knees, one nurse with palm up, the other with palm down, grasp wrists, lift with arms and shoulders, and remove to safety.

10. Double Cradle (to blanket)

    Unfold blanket on floor; same as No. 5 except that second nurse places knee nearest bed at right angles to patient's shoulder blades.

11. Double Kneel (to blanket)

    Unfold blanket on floor; same as No. 6, with one nurse at chest, the other at knees.

Three Nurses

12. Bed to Floor

    No. 1 grips just below and just above patient's knees; No. 2 grips patient just above and below waist, No. 3 grips upper back and shoulders. Pull patient to edge of bed; lift

Exhibit B continued

POLICY

Santa Monica Hospital Medical Center	POLICY NUMBER 6.7
	FUNCTIONAL AREA Safety & Disaster Hospital Wide
	PAGE 4 OF 5

SUBJECT: EMERGENCY REMOVAL OF PATIENTS	EFFECTIVE DATE Form: 5/78 Rev: 10/80
	APPROVED

in unison; then turn patient on side so patient is carried facing bearers on bearers' chests. Transport from room feet first, if possible. To lower patient: All three bearers drop to one knee (placing knee on floor) nearest patient's feet in unison and lower patient. Nurse at head of patient gives commands.

13. From Bed to Litter or Stretcher (right angle)
Same as No. 12, but patient on stretcher or litter.

14. From Bed to Blanket (triple kneel)
Same as No. 6 (kneel drop) and No. 11 (double kneel).

Four Nurses

15. Floor to Litter or Stretcher

Three nurses drop on knee, one placing knee nearest to patient's feet on floor; pick up patient as in No. 12; however, fourth nurse kneels opposite middle nurse and also grips below and above waist. All rise together in unison, turning patient on side as in No. 12. No. 1 nurse steps out and prepares litter or stretcher upon which remaining three nurses place patient as in No. 12.

16. Floor to Stretcher

Same as in No. 15. However, patient is lifted only knee high and then is allowed to rest on knees of first three nurses while nurse No. 4 steps out and prepares stretcher for patient.

Six Nurses

17. For Broken Back, Neck, or Pelvis

Three nurses on each side of bed, or if on floor, kneel on one knee nearest patient's feet on floor; two nurses at patient's head form cup behind head of patient by each nurse gripping own left wrist with right hand. Left hand will grip the other nurse's right wrist. Remaining hands of these nurses and the hands of other nurses are then to be placed alternatingly on each side of patient's back and worked under patient's body toward the spine area. All nurses lift together on command and place patient on litter, stiff stretcher, or blanket covered boards, by method outlined in No. 12.

Exhibit B continued

POLICY

Santa Monica	POLICY NUMBER 6.7

Santa Monica Hospital Medical Center

	POLICY NUMBER 6.7
	FUNCTIONAL Safety & Disaster
	AREA Hospital Wide
	PAGE 4 OF 5
SUBJECT:	EFFECTIVE Form: 5/78 Rev: 10/80
EMERGENCY REMOVAL OF PATIENTS	DATE
	APPROVED

Stretcher or Litter Carry

Stretchers or litters can be transported by two or four people. Bearers should walk out of step, if possible; i.e., persons or person in front should begin walking with left foot, persons or person at rear should begin with right foot, or vice versa. Patients should be transported feet first, if possible. Army type stretchers can be used. Poles in blankets can be utilized. Blankets with edges rolled make excellent stretchers, especially for negotiating stairs, fire escapes, or elevators.

Responsibility for review and revision of this policy has been assigned to

REVIEWED: _____ DATE: _____

REVIEWED: _____ DATE: _____

REVIEWED: _____ DATE: _____

REVIEWED: _____ DATE: _____

Source: Reprinted by permission from the *Disaster Plan Policy* of Santa Monica Hospital Medical Center, Santa Monica, Cal.

Appendix 4–F

Exhibit A: Disaster Preparedness

ST. ELIZABETH'S HOSPITAL

DEPARTMENTAL MANUAL

DIRECTIVE NO: 10-4500

EFFECTIVE DATE: September 8, 19

PAGE: 1 of 3

DIVISION: Disaster Preparedness

SECTION: Severe Weather

SUBJECT: Severe Weather

The Chicago Area can be subjected to a wide variety of severe weather conditions ranging from high winds, thunderstorms, tornados, and heavy snow. The purpose of this plan is to provide guidance when severe weather conditions are present.

Tornados

Definitions:

Tornado Watch: Issued for a period of several hours to warn a large area to the possibility of tornados.

Tornado Warning: Issued for a period of two hours or less when there is a high probability the area will be affected by a tornado. When issued, it may be based on visual sightings of tornados.

Tornado Alert: Announced only when there is impending danger to the area. It's often issued with a tornado warning.

Procedures

1. Notification of a tornado watch, warning or alert will be received by:

   News media, i.e., radio and television
   Police radio
   Weather radio

147

Exhibit A continued

DIRECTIVE NO: 10-4500   Page 2 of 3
SUBJECT: Severe Weather

2. When the notification is received, the administrator or designated representative shall be notified.
3. The individual contacting the administrator or designated representative shall request permission to implement the severe weather plan.
4. After approval has been received, the nursing supervisor and switchboard shall be notified of the plan implementation.

   A. The nursing supervisor shall contact all nursing units and the Professional Plaza as quickly as possible.

   1. All shades and drapes are to be pulled shut.
   2. Patients sitting next to the window shall be moved.
   3. The blinds in the Professional Plaza window shall be lowered and closed.

   B. Evacuation to the corridor shall not be accomplished until instructed to do so.
   C. All personnel should remain calm.
   D. There shall be no announcement over the public address system.
   E. Switchboard will contact *all* nonnursing departments.

5. When the danger is passed, the switchboard will be instructed to announce: "Resume normal activities." This announcement is to be made twice.
6. If St. Elizabeth's is struck by a tornado, the mass casualty plan will be implemented.
7. The engineer on duty will remain in the boiler room and will be prepared to shut down the boilers in the event a tornado strikes the hospital.
8. Maintenance and male housekeeping personnel on duty will report to security for assignment.

Thunderstorms and High Winds

1. Notification that thunderstorms and high winds are in the area shall be received by:

   News Media, i.e., radio and television
   Police Radio
   Weather Radio

2. When this warning has been received, the administrator or designated representative shall be notified and permission requested to activate the severe weather plan.

   A. The nursing supervisor and switchboard shall be notified.
   B. Switchboard will notify all nonnursing departments including the Professional Plaza.
   C. The nursing supervisor shall contact all nursing units.

   1. All shades and drapes are to be pulled shut.
   2. Patients sitting near the window shall be moved.
   3. The blinds in the Professional Plaza windows shall be lowered and closed.

Exhibit A continued

DIRECTIVE NO: 10-4500   Page   3   of   3
SUBJECT: Severe Weather

D.   The engineer on duty will remain in the boiler room and await further
instructions.
E.   Maintenance and male housekeeping personnel on duty will report to the security
shift supervisor for assignment.
F.   Security will secure all doors leading to the outside except the emergency room
entrance.
G.   When the danger is passed, switchboard will be instructed to announce: "Resume
normal activities." This announcement shall be made twice.

Heavy Snow

1.   Maintenance personnel are responsible for snow removal.
2.   After normal duty hours when the snow reaches a depth of ½ inch, the security shift
supervisor shall notify the maintenance supervisor, who shall contact the snow
removal teams.
3.   Security shall assist in the snow removal process by closing portions of the parking lot
and street so the snow team can remove snow as quickly as possible.
4.   If the snow becomes extremely heavy during normal duty hours, the administrator or
designated representative may declare a "snow day" and all nonessential personnel
may be sent home. The discussion as to who will go home will be made by the
individual supervisor.
5.   When a snow day is declared, the Director of Housekeeping Services will initiate a
bed availability inventory of the hospital and Margaritis Hall. This list, when
complete, is to be given to the administrator or designated representative.
6.   This list is to be used to assign sleeping accommodations when personnel and/or
visitors cannot go home because of the snow.
7.   Assignment of beds will be made by the administrator or designated representative.

Source: Reprinted with permission from the *Disaster Manual* of St. Elizabeth's Hospital,
Chicago, 1980.

Exhibit B: Saint Joseph Medical Center Bomb Threat Procedure

PURPOSE

Because of the alarming increase in frequency of property destruction and threats of such activity, it has become necessary to establish a Center position on prevention and clearly defined remedial steps to such action. The intent of this protocol is to appropriately prevent death or injury to patients and personnel or Medical Center property damage. It is the express purpose of these procedures to establish guidelines to be followed in the event of a bomb threat, explosion, or discovery of an explosive or incendiary device.

Due to the operational nature of the Medical Center and its facilities, which are open to the public, it is difficult to formulate a plan of action to fit each location. Therefore, we must rely upon each department and its employees to be informed and to report immediately any unusual person, activity, or object. A chain of command must be established within each department of the Medical Center to ensure prompt and intelligent action in the event of such an emergency.

The Burbank Police and Fire Departments will respond upon request, conduct a preliminary investigation, and take such action as dictated by the circumstances. However, they will not assume authority for the order of evacuation. This responsibility shall rest with the Administrator or designated alternate.

EXPLOSIVE DEVICES

The homemade bomb is usually one of two basic types. These are described as the open bomb and the concealed or disguised bomb. No effort is made to conceal the nature of the open type bomb. It is usually composed of one or more sticks of dynamite tied together and fitted with a safety fuse and blasting cap. It may consist of a short length of pipe, filled with an explosive, and capped at both ends with a piece of safety fuse protruding from a hole drilled in one of the caps. Sometimes a plastic substance having the appearance and consistency of putty is used. This material may be used in an open type bomb that is detonated by an explosive cap attached to electrical or safety fuse.

Explosive devices may be disguised or concealed in many ways. The most frequently used are shoeboxes, briefcases, and lunchboxes.

Exhibit B continued

PROCEDURE

Should a Medical Center employee receive a bomb threat call, he should remain as calm as possible and try to gain the maximum information from the caller. The number of incidents in which a bomb has actually been placed has increased, and it can no longer be assumed that the call is a hoax.

Response:

PBX—a person receiving telephone bomb threat.

Action Sequence

A. Immediately upon receiving any bomb threats via telephone, the exact time shall be logged. All actions taken by PBX, such as notification of key personnel, shall be logged and timed until she is notified that the situation is cleared and all departments are back to normal. Particular attention shall be made to the exact words used by the caller. ANY INFORMATION OBTAINED FROM THE CALLER IS OF THE UTMOST IMPORTANCE! (refer to PBX "Bomb Threat Checklist"). [Appendix 4–F, Exhibit C]

The following questions should be asked:

1. What building or office is the bomb in?
2. Where in the building or office (inside, outside, roof, basement, etc.)
3. What does it look like? (box, suitcase, pipe, shoebox, etc.)
4. What type of explosive used?
5. When is it set to go off? (exact time and date)

Some other suggestions that might help:

1. Pay particular attention to any strange or peculiar background noises.
2. Listen closely to the voice—male or female; age; voice quality—accent or speech impediment. Record every word and impression immediately and notify the Administrator or designated alternate.

B. If threat is received on a weekday between 8 a.m. and 5 p.m.:

1. Contact the Administrator or designated alternate and advise them of the situation and stand by for instructions.
2. Contact the Security Department and advise of the situation.
3. Notify the Director of Security.

C. If threat is received on weekends and/or after 5 p.m.:

1. Notify Supervisor in Charge.
2. Contact the Administrator or the Administrator-on-call at his residence, advise him of the situation, and stand by for instructions.
3. Contact the Security Department and advise of the situation.
4. Notify the Director of Security at his residence.

Exhibit B continued

Response:

Administrator
Associate Administrator
Administrative Alternate
Director of Security

Action Sequence

A. Upon being notified that the Medical Center has received such a bomb threat, the Administrator or designated alternate will initiate the following:

1. Will make all decisions regarding searches, key personnel notification, outside agency notification, possible command post locations, evacuations, and other decisions pertaining to the bomb threat incident.
2. Should a general recall of Medical Center personnel be ordered by Administration, the Disaster Personnel Notification Procedure will be used.
3. If a bomb is found, the following shall apply:

   a. Order evacuation of all personnel from the area. Ensure all personnel remain at a safe distance. It should be noted that a distance of 1,000 feet away from the concerned area is considered a safe distance.
   b. Inspect the area to assure that the area has been completely evacuated.
   c. Make sure that no person touches a suspect object/device or anything attached to it. DO NOT ATTEMPT TO MOVE, COVER, OR JAR IT. LEAVE IT ALONE!
   d. Have personnel standing by in the nearest lobby or entrance to guide and assist the police department bomb disposal squad.
   e. Have preselected personnel at strategic locations to prevent unauthorized persons from entering the area.

B. In case an incendiary device is ignited:

1. The Medical Center Fire and Internal Disaster Plan and its procedures will be activated. Each department will perform its duties as outlined in these procedures.

C. In case of a bomb explosion:

1. The Administrator, after appraising the extent of damage and casualties, shall utilize the Disaster and Mass Casualty Plan and its procedures.
2. Triage teams along with available physicians and nurses shall be directed to an area not affected by the bomb blast.
3. Guard the explosion scene from unauthorized persons pending an investigation by law enforcement and safety personnel.
4. Have preselected personnel assigned to strategic locations to prevent unauthorized persons from entering the affected area.
5. Give the ALL CLEAR and notify concerned departments to return to normal operations.

Exhibit B continued

Response:

Administration
Nursing Department

Action Sequence

A. In case of a bomb located on a patient floor:

1. If it is determined that the threat of a bomb in the Medical Center is fact, particularly if determined to be on a patient floor, Administration is to advise the Nursing Service to proceed with the following precautionary measures:

   a. Head nurses must get patients away from all windows and attempt to cover those windows with blankets in order to prevent flying glass.
   b. If the identified device is located in a patient area and patients cannot be moved, attempt to provide a minimum of two walls between the suspected bomb and the patient.
   c. Open all doors within the suspected area to allow the force of an explosion to be dissipated.
   d. Do not pull a fire alarm or otherwise alarm the patients. Act as casual as possible and attempt to have a reasonable explanation for the functions being performed.
   e. If evacuation is advised by the police or fire department, the Administrator will advise all concerned departments regarding the evacuation.

Response:

Director of Security
Security Officers

Action Sequence

A. As soon as the Department of Security has been advised of a bomb threat, the following procedures are to be implemented:

1. All doors providing ingress and egress in the Medical Center will be secured.
2. A systematic search of the Medical Center will begin immediately by the duty officer.
3. The security officer recall plan will be immediately put into effect. Four reserve security officers will be called at their residences and given instructions to report at once.
4. If a bomb or a suspect device is located within the Medical Center or on its surrounding property, notification will immediately be sent to the Administration or designated alternate.
5. Police department members on the scene will notify their operations officer that a bomb has been found and they will notify other outside agencies as may be required.

Source: Reprinted with permission from the *Disaster Manual* of St. Joseph Medical Center, Burbank, Cal., 1983.

Appendix 4–F

Exhibit C: Bomb Threat Checklist

INSTRUCTIONS: LISTEN, DO NOT INTERRUPT THE CALLER EXCEPT TO ASK:

1. When will it go off? _____
2. Where is it planted? _____
3. What does it look like? _____
4. What floor is it on? _____
5. Why are you doing this? _____
6. Who are you? _____

Call Received By	Time of Call	Date

Description of Caller	Approximate Age of Caller
☐ Male ☐ Female ☐ Adult ☐ Juvenile	

VOICE CHARACTERISTICS		SPEECH		LANGUAGE	
☐ Loud	☐ Soft	☐ Fast	☐ Slow	☐ Excellent	☐ Good
☐ High Pitched	☐ Deep	☐ Distinct	☐ Distorted	☐ Fair	☐ Poor
☐ Raspy	☐ Pleasant	☐ Stutter	☐ Nasal	☐ Foul	☐ Other
☐ Intoxicated	☐ Other	☐ Slurred	☐ Precise		
		☐ Other _____		☐ Use of certain words or phrases	

ACCENT		MANNER		BACKGROUND NOISES	
☐ Local	☐ Not Local	☐ Calm	☐ Angry	☐ Office Machines	☐ Street Traffic
☐ Foreign	☐ Regional	☐ Rational	☐ Irrational	☐ Factory Machines	☐ Airplanes
☐ Race	☐ Other	☐ Coherent	☐ Incoherent	☐ Bedlam	☐ Trains
Explain _____		☐ Deliberate	☐ Emotional	☐ Animals	☐ Voices
_____		☐ Righteous	☐ Laughing	☐ Quiet	☐ Music
				☐ Mixed	☐ Party Atmosphere

ACTION TO TAKE IMMEDIATELY AFTER CALL—
1. Notify Security.
2. Notify your supervisor.
3. Write exact language of caller below.

_____

_____

_____

Appendix 4–F

Exhibit D: Earthquake Procedure

POLICY

Santa Monica Hospital Medical Center

POLICY NUMBER	9.1
FUNCTIONAL AREA	Safety & Disaster Hospital Wide
PAGE	1 OF 2

SUBJECT: EARTHQUAKE PROCEDURE	EFFECTIVE Form: 4/79 Rev: DATE APPROVED

Purpose:

The purpose of this procedure is to establish guidelines for employees to follow in the event of an earthquake. In order for it to be effective, *all* personnel must be familiar with its contents.

General Procedure:

Everyone's safety depends on each employee's remaining calm.
1. Remain calm. Do not panic or run through or outside the building. The great point of danger is just outside doorways and close to outer walls because of falling debris.
2. If you are in the building, remain where you are. If possible, take cover under desk, table or bench, or in doorways, hallways, or against inside walls. These areas are the most sound structurally during an earthquake.
3. Keep visitors, patients, and other employees out of stairwells and elevators. (The elevator system is equipped to shut down during an earthquake and open at the nearest floor.)
4. If you are outside, stay away from the building. Stay clear of walls, utility poles, downed wires, and trees.
5. The most important thing to remember is to remain calm. Reassure and assist patients and visitors. DO NOT ABANDON YOUR PATIENTS.
6. If possible, turn off utilities. Extinguish all smoking materials. Use good judgment.

In case of damage to:

A. Gas:
   1. Inspect for leaky pipes, by smell only.
   2. If you smell gas:
      a. Contact Engineering for immediate assistance.
      b. Open all windows and doors so gas can escape.
      c. Engineering will shut off the main valve.
      d. Notify PBX, which will in turn notify the gas company. Make sure you give the operator the exact location of the affected area.

155

Exhibit D continued

POLICY

Santa Monica
Hospital
Medical Center

POLICY NUMBER	9.1
FUNCTIONAL AREA	Safety & Disaster Hospital Wide
PAGE	2 OF 2

SUBJECT:	EFFECTIVE	Form: 4/79 Rev:
EARTHQUAKE PROCEDURE	DATE	
	APPROVED	

    B. Water:
        If pipes are broken, Engineering will shut off the main valves which bring water into the hospital.

    C. Electricity:
        The hospital is properly wired. Trouble is very unlikely. If there is a short circuit call Engineering for immediate assistance.

NOTE: Each department should evaluate its area and set up specific procedures to follow in the event of damage to utilities. This is particularly important for areas where gas of any kind is used.

7. If a fire occurs, follow *Fire Procedure.*
8. If evacuation is necessary, follow *Evacuation Procedure.*

Remember

If an earthquake occurs:

1. Remain calm.
2. Assure patients' safety. DO NOT ABANDON PATIENTS.
3. Do not try to leave or enter building.
4. Stay away from outer walls, windows, trees, utility poles, and downed wires.
5. Check utilities.
6. Use telephones only for emergency.
7. Above all, use *good judgment.*

Responsibility for review and revision of this policy has been assigned to

REVIEWED: _____ DATE: _____
REVIEWED: _____ DATE: _____
REVIEWED: _____ DATE: _____
REVIEWED: _____ DATE: _____

Source: Reprinted with permission from the *Disaster Plan Policy* of Santa Monica Hospital Medical Center, Santa Monica, Cal.

Chapter 5

Disaster Preparedness Training and Drills

Planning is worthless unless staff members understand the basic concepts of disaster response and can function appropriately in a disaster event.

Successful disaster preparedness begins with the Disaster Planning Committee and the Disaster Coordinator. When they enthusiastically support training and drills, employees also will become enthused and administrators will be more likely to allocate resources for training.

Training is a descriptive term for a range of instructional and experiential learning experiences. Some of these are formal classroom events with prepared curricula and materials; others are less formal, held at the worksite, and involve coaching and practice; still others are purely experiential—events of everyday life and during extraordinary circumstances (such as disaster).

TRAINING MODALITIES

Adults are less apt to resist training (and more likely to learn) if varied methods are used. The choice of one training modality over another depends on many variables, including the goals and objectives of the program, the audience mix, and situational factors such as personnel turnover rates and the amount of time since the last program. Table 5–1 details several training modalities.

Formal Classroom or Worksite Training

This type of training program utilizes formal didactic and/or experiential methods. Programs are scheduled for specific dates, times, and locales. Because disaster preparedness is not a topic in frequent demand, program planning should include preparation of publicity materials designed to encourage attendance. Even if attendance is mandatory, an attempt should be made to personalize invitations and stress the importance of participation.

Table 5–1 Training Modalities

Formal Classroom or Worksite Locations		Informal Worksite Locations
Didactic	**Experiential**	**Experiential**
• Lectures	• Simulation games	• Tabletop drills
• Panel presentations	• Case studies	• On-the-spot review drills
• Written materials	• Discussion and critique workshops	• Subelement drills
• Media: AV, TV/VCR	• Computer–assisted interactive problem solving	• Discussion groups
• Personal computer		• Critique sessions
	• Field trips, tours	• Facility critique
	• Dissemination of materials to worksites, e.g., disaster manuals, interesting journal articles	
	• Coordinated disaster exercises	

Training events have more emotional impact and their results are longer lasting if they are exciting. Motivational speakers, provocative simulation games, and case studies are alternatives to the traditional (and all too often boring) disaster preparedness lectures. One critical variable that affects the learning climate is the relative freedom of participants to share openly their expectations and experience, whether positive or negative. Lecture presentations that do not allow audience participation should be discouraged.

Handout materials are helpful if they relate to the theme or content of the program. However, distributing too much material will saturate the audience, and too many sensationalist articles will only titillate rather than instruct. Because there is a good deal of disaster literature, care should be taken to select items appropriate to the audience mix and program content for each specific presentation. Material distributed before a formal program and accompanied by a personal note from the Disaster Coordinator on its relevancy to the upcoming class may be a significant motivator.

Formal instruction also can take place at the worksite. The use of on-the-job settings lends reality to training content. Methods include demonstrating the use of equipment, computer-assisted learning, field trips and observations, and a host of other applications.

Informal Worksite Training

Frequent and varied training programs and drills with changing scenarios are a useful method for sustaining interest in disaster preparedness. While some of the programs involve structure, others do not. For instance, small group discussions of singular aspects of the disaster plan do not require much prior preparation, nor does the discussion. This setting encourages the free flow of questions and answers with unrestricted feedback. It stimulates involvement.

TRAINING CONCEPTS

While training and teaching both are educational processes, they are not synonymous. Teaching assumes *tabula rasa*—the concept of the learner as receptive but with a mental "blank slate." The role of the teacher is to "fill in the blanks." Training takes quite the opposite point of view. Training views the learner as an active, discerning partner, rather than a blank with no experience or expectation.

The most important consideration in disaster training is that it is first and foremost an adult education experience. Rather than the traditional didactic classroom event typical of much inservice education in health care, disaster training should incorporate instructional methods that involve the participants actively. The basic tenet of adult education is that participants bring a lifetime of experience and bias with them to every learning situation. Adult learners tend to acquire new skills most readily when ideas presented are linked to both their prior experience and to training events. Adults in general and health care personnel in particular tend to regard their own competence highly. Resistance to training diminishes and retention of new information and skills increases when they have the opportunity to critique the training event on their own and/or with their peers. Table 5–2 highlights differences between the concepts of teaching and training.

Any health educator who has taught a mandatory basic cardiopulmonary resuscitation (CPR) course to physicians knows firsthand the resistance and skepticism of most participants. Resistant attitudes often change if participants are given the opportunity to discuss the experience. This situation in many respects is similar to the way personnel respond to mandatory disaster training programs.

Disaster training can be unsettling. Fear, anxiety, and discomfort may develop, creating a significant learning barrier. But the intent of training is to reduce, rather than create, barriers. Structuring training events in such a way that participants are able to share experience and feelings while at the same time building upon their existing competencies will be helpful. Negative feedback should be avoided. Successful disaster training recognizes that:

Table 5–2 Selected Differences between Teaching and Training Concepts

Views of	Traditional Teaching Approach	Training as Adult Education Approach
Learner	Student (passive child)	Participant (active adult)
Learning setting	Primarily classroom	Classroom and nonclassroom settings
Learning climate	Reactive	Interactive
Methods	Didactic (prescriptive, "teacher tell")	Socratic (trainer helps participants discover "truth" themselves)
Knowledge	Knosis (traditional medical model: teacher diagnoses students' needs and knows what is "best")	Collaborative

- Trainees filter every training experience and activity through their own perceptions, regardless of how much importance others attribute to the training.
- Adults learn by doing, so training should involve participants as much as possible in discussion, analysis, and dialogue with presenters.
- Nothing is sacrosanct; if a participant knows of another way to do something, it should be considered valid (at least for discussion purposes) and certainly not rejected out of hand.
- Participants learn as much from talking with one another as they do from listening to experts.

Figure 5–1 depicts the complex factors affecting learners in any training event.

BARRIERS TO TRAINING

Disaster preparedness training faces an array of constraints. These predispose the training effort to failure, so trainers should be aware of them. Many of these barriers have similar causes and require a similar approach.

Figure 5–1 Selected Variables That Can Influence Training

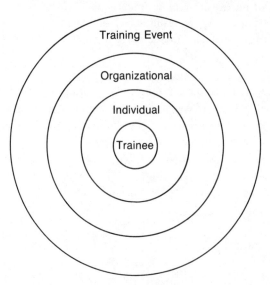

Training Event Variables	*Organizational Variables*	*Individual Variables*
• Trainer behavior, affect, language • Training methods • Training site logistics • Apparent importance of training content • Opportunity to practice and/or critique training experience • Whether training is voluntary or mandatory	• Prevailing norms • Peer influence • Professional standards • Opportunity to apply training immediately on the job • Rewards for participation and for new learning and behavior change • Penalties for nonparticipation	• Self-recognition of need • Prior formal education and training experiences • Psychological needs to belong, compete, perform • Value ascribed to peer, superior, subordinate expectations • Ability to acquire and retain new information and skills • Willingness to change • Life experience

Personal Relevance

People will not participate enthusiastically in planning if they consider the planned-for events unlikely to occur or if the events are felt to be of no personal relevance.

This basic impediment to disaster preparedness often is overlooked. However, it creates lack of interest in training, reduces the participation required in drill planning and response, and can result in lack of plan revision when that becomes necessary. Strategies that can be used to overcome this problem include:

- Holding frequent discussions related to both personal preparedness and facility preparedness; these can take place during staff meetings.
- Disseminating materials produced by community, state, and federal planning agencies; these can be placed in staff communication manuals, on bulletin boards, and in department mail boxes.
- Holding informal discussions on how people react to disaster planning, prewarnings, and prior evacuation; this should cover recent disasters in the community and the potential for others to occur.
- Involving staff in planning for training sessions and drills.

Disinterest and Stagnancy

Disaster preparedness fades quickly as immediate problems take precedence. This is a widespread phenomenon. The day-to-day demands of a complex medical facility easily preempt disaster preparedness training plans. When drills and other events are held they often are critiqued poorly, and what is learned from them (such as personnel interface, patient flow problems, etc.) is not used to revise the *Disaster Manual*. Once the disaster planning process is completed and the manual written, stagnancy can occur all too easily. This has a deleterious effect on the morale of everyone involved, and is in itself evidence of denial.

Other strategies for overcoming the problem of "preparedness fade" include:

- Designating a full-time disaster coordinator whose primary responsibility is disaster planning and training.
- Encouraging supervisory personnel to serve as role models for a "get prepared and stay prepared" philosophy. An important aim of any preparedness training effort should be to prepare senior and middle management personnel to carry out various elements of the training plan. Creative ways for doing this include tabletop drills* at management meetings, monthly review of disaster preparedness progress at management meetings, and biannual training preparedness programs for managers.

---

*Tabletop drill is the term used to describe a paper/pencil training exercise. For example, instead of enacting a referral of well walk-in disaster patients from triage to the correct receiving unit, the tabletop drill exercise would pose the question and require a response, either verbal or written.

- Recognizing the time managers and staff members spend on disaster preparedness. Recognition can be provided as financial compensation, "comp" time, and substitution of disaster preparedness activities for other responsibilities.

Integration into Regular Operations

Preparedness is likely to fail if it is not made a routine part of facility operation. Developing competence takes time. While many skills must be learned, the most important of these are judgment and decision making. These can be developed only with practice. One commonly held but inaccurate assumption is that knowledge of basic nursing practice and patient management are sufficient for effective disaster response. The reality is that disaster response requires the modification of existing skills and daily patient care routines.

Annual or biannual drills will not establish or maintain competency. Preparedness requires new skills and their reinforcement through considerable practice. Passive activities such as reading a manual will not improve disaster judgment skills. Instead, preparedness should emphasize action activities carefully planned to promote the development of adaptive behavior during a disaster.

Strategies for overcoming this barrier include:

- Providing classroom instruction in disaster principles. Classroom training should be followed with drills that reinforce the concepts presented in the classroom and that provide an opportunity for active participation.
- Accompanying training with testing. Some standard must be used to determine the extent of training needed and whether or not the training provided succeeded in meeting that need.
- Using staff members in the review of standards for disaster response, for plan revision, and for the organization of drill exercises.
- Holding drills in logical progression. A multifacility/agency exercise with mock casualties would be counterproductive for an institution that only recently has revised its plan and whose staff has not been trained yet in its implementation.
- Scheduling controlled drills frequently. These can include paper drills, tabletop drills, and subelement drills (see discussion later in this chapter).

Barriers to successful preparedness training are not insurmountable. The extent to which any facility elects to prepare its personnel is limited only by fear, philosophy, and sometimes funding. The vital point is that unless recognized and addressed purposefully, these barriers can turn a preparedness program into a failure.

DISASTER TRAINING

Effective response to a disaster depends upon realistic planning, available resources, and trained personnel. Facility employees must know what is expected of them and how their roles interrelate with others. Without adequate training, role ambiguity and conflict are inevitable. Untrained workers in a disaster exacerbate problems and increase risks for victims and rescuers alike. An accounting clerk who is assigned to the role of messenger in a disaster is as significant to facility response as is a registered nurse assigned to the Major Treatment Area, and must know the role and function of the messenger in a disaster.

Health care staff members and other personnel may resist disaster training because they are uncomfortable with the topic and what it implies for them and their families. They also may resist because they fear loss of status, independence, and/or freedom of action.

For example, a small, Midwest facility found itself ill prepared to handle casualties from a bus accident. An unexpected problem emerged when one of the two plant engineers on duty refused to function as a security officer. In the postdisaster critique, the engineer said: "I thought I should stay near the boiler in case more heat was needed. Besides, security is not my job and I shouldn't be doing it!"

Preparedness training, for the most part, should be mandatory for everyone— including attending staff physicians. Unfortunately, concern about physicians' reaction has caused many trainers to avoid mandating their participation. In some areas of the country, local medical associations are very supportive and encourage their members to attend disaster-related training programs. Some associations sponsor disaster training as continuing education events; others sponsor programs for clinicians whether or not they are members of the association.

Once the disaster plan has been developed and/or revised, all personnel must be trained appropriately. The term "appropriate" is significant here; clinical nurses will require training different from housekeeping personnel, the needs of security personnel will differ from the business office, etc. Preparing individuals to perform expected roles is the next step after the plan is completed and a manual is distributed.

Preparedness training requires careful planning and is most cost effective when programs are scheduled on a yearly basis. The following sequence is suggested:

1. assess training needs
2. develop a comprehensive 12-month training plan
3. develop training goals and objectives for each program in the training plan
4. identify and select training resources for the programs
5. develop content for each program
6. identify the approximate number of participants for each training program
7. organize programs with a mix of training methods.

1. Assess Training Needs

Learning needs can be identified in a variety of ways: surveying with a questionnaire, evaluating responses to a skills inventory, brainstorming with groups of personnel, and trainer assessment of personnel performance during drills. Examples of a questionnaire, skills inventory, and observation rating forms are presented in Exhibits 5–1, 5–2, and 5–3.

2. Develop a 12-Month Training Plan

Exhibit 5–4 is an example of a 12-month disaster preparedness training plan for a 350-bed acute care facility. A 12-month plan allows sufficient time for scheduling individual events and advertising them, reserving classroom space as needed, identifying and confirming speakers, scheduling personnel attendance, and developing the training curricula.

3. Develop Goals and Objectives

At least two goals should be developed for each program to specify what accomplishments will be expected. For example:

The general orientation program on disaster preparedness will:

- provide all personnel with an overview of the hospital's role in disaster response
- use lecture, discussion, and question/answer techniques to present disaster preparedness concepts

Once goals are stated in writing, the next step is to develop behavior-oriented objectives that specify what behavior changes will be expected as a result of the learning experience. Development of behavioral objectives should be done for all training programs (see Exhibit 5–5).

The behavioral objectives should be action oriented and measurable. Terms such as "appreciate" or "have an awareness of" are not measurable and as such cannot be used to assess change in skills or knowledge.

4. Identify and Select Training Resources

Training resources include classroom space, audiovisual equipment, handout materials, and training personnel. Training personnel include experts in disaster response who may have to be recruited from outside the facility as well as group

Exhibit 5–1 Questionnaire To Survey Personnel Disaster Training Learning Needs

We need your help to determine the aspects of disaster preparedness that you would like to learn more about and whether there are skills and abilities you wish to improve. Please answer the following questions. Thank you for your help. There is no need to sign this form.

Please read the list below carefully. For each item check one of the three answers:

        YES for each item you wish to learn more about
        NO   for any item that does not interest you
        ?   for any item about which you are uncertain

	Yes	No	?
1. Where to find my unit manual	☐	☐	☐
2. What paperwork is involved in a disaster	☐	☐	☐
3. How we will be notified of a disaster while at work	☐	☐	☐
4. How personnel assignments will be made when a disaster is declared	☐	☐	☐
5. How our facility defines a disaster	☐	☐	☐
6. Where the Personnel Pool will be located	☐	☐	☐
7. Who will be in charge of my unit during a disaster	☐	☐	☐
8. What the public address announcement will be	☐	☐	☐
9. What to do in case of a fire in our hospital	☐	☐	☐
10. What to do in case of a bomb threat	☐	☐	☐
11. How communications will be managed in our hospital	☐	☐	☐
12. How to evacuate patients from our unit	☐	☐	☐
13. How Triage will function	☐	☐	☐
14. Where the Major Treatment Area will be	☐	☐	☐
15. What the Command Post will do	☐	☐	☐
16. What plant engineering will do if we have a disaster affecting our facility's structure	☐	☐	☐

ADDITIONAL ITEMS THAT INTEREST ME BUT ARE NOT INCLUDED ABOVE:

A. _____

B. _____

C. _____

Exhibit 5–2 Example of Skills Inventory of Disaster Response for RNs

SPECIFIED SKILLS FOR RNs IN A DISASTER RESPONSE	RATINGS Codes: 1—needs complete training 2—needs some improvement 3—current performance satisfactory		
Ability to:	*1*	*2*	*3*
1. Locate unit manual			
2. Locate Disaster Action Cards			
3. Initiate staff callback			
4. Report a disaster			
5. Complete disaster-related paper work			
6. Determine capacity of unit			
7. Identify patients for evacuation/transfer/ discharge			
8. Initiate physical call for patient removal from unit			
9. Make staff assignment			
10. Identify unit equipment/ supply/personnel needs			
11. Etc.			

discussion leaders or lecturers drawn from the institution itself. If the training event involves mock casualties, makeup specialists may have to be employed.

5. Develop Content for Each Program

Content should be based on program goals and objectives, on behavioral objectives, and on time constraints. While content is being developed, attention also should be given to how behavioral change will be measured. An objective examination containing multiple-choice questions is helpful, as is a participant workbook. Workbook responses to case studies, for example, can be used to indicate learning as well as training needs.

Exhibit 5–6 is an excerpt from a multiple-choice posttraining objective test.

6. Identify Number of Program Participants

The appropriate mix of employees is important. There are occasions when participants should include physicians, staff, and supervisory personnel; there also are times when this mix is inappropriate. Appropriateness depends on the goals of

Exhibit 5–3 Example: Observer Rating Form—Learning Needs

DATE _____ TIME _____ LOCATION _____
OBSERVER _____

	Yes	No	?
Disaster Concepts			
Can staff define "disaster"?	☐	☐	☐
Do personnel know how the hospital plan interrelates with the community plan?	☐	☐	☐
Do personnel know what the disaster philosophy of the facility is?	☐	☐	☐
Are they aware of how physicians and prehospital providers will function in an external disaster?	☐	☐	☐
Do they know what to do if they are at home when a disaster is declared?	☐	☐	☐
Disaster Plan Implementation			
Do personnel know how to verify a disaster if they receive initial notification from outside the facility?	☐	☐	☐
Do they know how the personnel on duty will be notified?	☐	☐	☐
Do they know what FIRST ACTION they should take upon public address announcement of a disaster?	☐	☐	☐
Do they know how to determine need for more staff on their unit?	☐	☐	☐
Do they know how to obtain staffing supplements for their unit?	☐	☐	☐
Do they know how to complete a unit status report?	☐	☐	☐
Disaster Plan Operation			
Can they locate Triage?	☐	☐	☐
Major Treatment?	☐	☐	☐
Delayed Treatment?	☐	☐	☐
Command Post?	☐	☐	☐
Do they know how they will be identified while working in the facility during a disaster?	☐	☐	☐
Can they define "Immediate" and "Delayed" casualties?	☐	☐	☐
Do they know what their unit will be responsible for during a disaster?	☐	☐	☐

Comments: _____

the training. Goals and objectives also influence group size. Small groups are better for hands-on practice events held in a conference room or classroom setting, while formal instructional presentations and panel discussions are more suitable for larger groups.

Exhibit 5–4 Example of 12–Month Training Plan

Training Needs / Priorities:	Probable Duration	Schedule (month)	Participants (approximate number)				
			Ancillary Depts.	Admin. Depts.	Med./ Surg.	Med. Staff	Disaster Committee
1. Disaster Manual	2 hours	Jan.-Mar.	212	141	314	60	
2. Role of Nursing in: triage mobilization and functions, casualty management, victim education, victim orientation	8 hours	Mar. and Oct.	25	10	125	15	
3. Fire drill, simulated patient education	two 2-hour events	June and Nov.	35	22	110	15	
4. JCAH requirements	1 hour	June		22			15
5. Crisis counseling methods	6 hours	Sept.	25	10	125	15	
6. Psychosocial aspects of disaster	6 hours	Oct.	25	10	110		15
7. Facility integrity after earthquake	4 hours	Nov.	15				

Exhibit 5–5 Examples of Behavioral Objectives for a Disaster Preparedness
Program

At the conclusion of this program, the learner will:

1. define "disaster"
2. list three categories of patient-generating incidents
3. identify at least four actions to take immediately after a disaster occurs to protect self and
   family
4. describe the institution's disaster philosophy
5. discuss the function of a facility disaster plan
6. identify where the disaster plan for the participant's unit is stored
7. explain the difference between an internal and an external disaster
8. identify the major components of the *Disaster Manual*:

   a. Command Post
   b. Triage Area
   c. Personnel Callback
   d. Personnel Assignment/Pool
   e. Public Relations/Media Relations
   f. Security
   g. Major/Minor Treatment Areas

9. describe "disaster alert" public address announcement for both "standby" and "mobilize" alerts

If small group sessions are to be held, it may be necessary to plan each session
for different times so that all personnel in various classifications can attend. For
instance, if 60 nurses are to participate in a small group meeting, as many as four
different sessions of the same program will have to be scheduled (15 nurses × 4
= N60). In general, holding the same program on at least two different dates and
times will allow the most flexibility for staff attendance.

7. Organize Each Training Program

Factors to consider in organizing training include scheduling suitable training
sites, scheduling meals and/or refreshments, and ordering sufficient numbers of
handout materials. If a syllabus is to be distributed, sufficient preparation time
should be allocated so that all supplemental materials can be included.

If at all possible, a variety of training methods should be used. In general, adult
learners will be less resistant if given the opportunity for dialogue with one another
and with the trainers. Training methods should be planned to stimulate participant
involvement. The basic key to a meaningful learning experience is the use of
several different methods in a single program. Examples of methods useful in
disaster preparedness training are listed in Table 5–3.

Exhibit 5–6 Excerpt from a Posttraining Exam

POSTCOURSE EXAM

NAME _____
DATE _____

Please circle the letter preceding the *most* appropriate answer to each statement.

1. A hospital plan will be most effective if it is:

   A. tested with realism
   B. developed by the triad of Hospital Administration, Nursing Administration, and Medical Staff Chief
   C. revised at least once a year
   D. tested systematically and revised with input from drill participants

2. The role of hospital Disaster Coordinator includes:

   A. revising the general hospital plan
   B. coordinating drills and educating staff
   C. performing individual department prospective critiques
   D. moderating postdrill general critique sessions

3. Conduct a drill only:

   A. after all staff members are thoroughly trained
   B. when moulaged victims are available
   C. when it is a complete surprise
   D. the plan is developed and you know what you want to evaluate

4. Once critique of a drill is held, the next action is to:

   A. provide feedback on the critique immediately to all participants
   B. establish problem priority and a timetable for action
   C. file the critique report for JCAH review
   D. advise staff of the problems and schedule a drill

A detailed discussion of 12 of these methods is presented in Appendix 5–A, at the end of this chapter.

ATTENDANCE AT TRAINING EVENTS

Attendance at preparedness educational events must be mandatory. All personnel must know what is expected of them. There are advantages and disadvantages to a mandatory training philosophy, however. The primary advantage is that

Table 5–3 Disaster Preparedness Training Methods

Action Methods	Demonstration Methods	Didactic Methods
• Simulations	• Role Play	• Lecture
• Drills	• Multimedia:	• Panel
• Rehearsals	VCR	• Symposium
• On-the-Job:	TV	• Forum
Coaching	Audio tapes	• Incident Process
Practice	Movies	• Conference
Job Rotation	• Charts, Diagrams	
	• Written Materials	
	• Case Studies	

everyone will be exposed to the same information and have the same opportunities for practice. The disadvantages are:

1. A mandatory program contradicts a fundamental tenet of adult education, which is the assumption that adults are self-motivated to learn. Mandatory attendance almost always creates barriers to learning.
2. Mandatory programs usually are held during normal work hours, necessitating extra personnel costs for shift coverage of those who attend. If personnel attend on their days off, regular or overtime wages may have to be allocated. Either way, mandatory education requires budgeting for extra personnel costs.

Scheduling several meetings of the same program for different dates and times can minimize the need to cover worker shifts and provide individual choice within the mandatory requirement.

The Disaster Coordinator should have primary responsibility for coordinating training content and scheduling as well as for tracking and tabulating both personnel attendance and subjective evaluations of training events. Inasmuch as disaster preparedness has life-and-death implications, the facility must know with a relatively high degree of certainty which employees attend, even though attendance obviously is not an indicator of learning retention or skills acquisition.

TYPES OF TRAINING PROGRAMS

At a minimum, four basic types of training should be scheduled annually:

1. Core Disaster Training Programs
2. Quarterly Core Programs

3. Training-of-Trainer Programs
4. Follow-Up Department/Work Unit Training Programs

Figure 5–2 is an example of the sequencing of these programs in an acute care facility. The program content is based upon needs identified in the early phase of program planning.

Core Training Program

This generic program provides disaster response concepts, philosophy, and policy training for personnel at all levels. The core program is a basic orientation that establishes a "disaster mind-set." Exhibit 5–7 is an example of a curriculum outline for this type of program.

The sample program shown in Exhibit 5–7 has two general objectives: (1) to introduce learners to disaster preparedness concepts and (2) to present key elements of disaster response specific to the facility.

Whoever develops and conducts the original program must be knowledgeable about disaster theory and facility response. Trainers for the core program become role models, particularly for supervisors and managers. Skill in leading groups and in utilizing various presentation methods is essential. Unit supervisors who will be expected to maintain unit preparedness must have group-leading and training

---

Figure 5–2 Example of Program Sequence for a 12–Month Training Plan

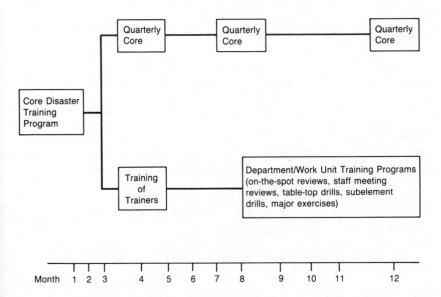

Exhibit 5–7 Example of Curriculum Outline for One-Day Core Program

Time (Minutes)	Outline	Method
20	A. Introduction 1. Purpose and objectives of this program 2. Pretest 3. Purpose of emergency preparedness	1. Lecture 2. Hand out/collect 3. Lecture
60	B. Definition of a disaster: Myths and Realities 1. Definition/categories of disasters 2. Disasters to which this community is at risk 3. What federal, state, and local governments will do in response 4. Planning for self and family	1. Agree/disagree pyramid 2. Lecture
Break, 15 minutes		
60	C. Medical Center Planning 1. Our disaster philosophy, goals, and objectives 2. "Internal" vs. "external" disasters, definition 3. How our plan was developed 4. What the plan looks like, where it can be found 5. Components of our plan 6. Notification system for disasters involving our hospital	1. Symposium 2. 16mm film 3. Subgroups reacting to film
Lunch Break, 45 minutes		
60	D. Large-scale disasters 1. How our hospital will respond 2. Postdisaster considerations	1. Overhead projector 2. Q & A 3. Handouts
Break, 15 minutes		
40	E. Training and drills 1. Why, when, where, how will we train? 2. Purpose of drills 3. Description of a subelement drill 4. Description of a moulaged drill exercise	1. Lecture 2. Slides
30	F. Summary/questions/answers 1. The "disaster mentality," denial, and motivation to be prepared	1. Three-minute audio tape 2. Q & A

Exhibit 5–7 continued

Time *(Minutes)*	*Outline*	*Method*
15	2. Summary of class content 3. Posttest 4. Adjourn	1. Lecture 2. Hand out/collect
285 minutes		

skills as well. Some facilities use specialists on an ad hoc basis, either to coach their own disaster training personnel or to participate as resource persons in training events.

Core programs are usually didactic and presented to large groups. The first core program each year is likely to have the largest attendance, with fewer participants at subsequent quarterly core programs. The latter are designed for new employees and tenured staff returning for review.

Core programs usually are structured as auditorium or classroom presentations, in part because audiovisual aids such as slides and/or transparencies require forward-facing seat arrangements. Figure 5–3 is an example of a slide used to illustrate a core program lecture.

Auditorium seating does not preclude opportunities to use various training methods to stimulate the audience. A useful technique for helping participants to feel at ease quickly and for generating enthusiasm is an "icebreaker" that involves the audience in the topic. Exhibit 5–8 is an example of an icebreaker handout.

After the handout is distributed, the audience members are asked to take no longer than five minutes to look over the list and then, as individuals, to check whether they agree or disagree with each statement. They then are asked to quickly form random groups of four to eight persons to reach a consensus on their agreement or disagreement with each statement. The trainer stops the discussion after a reasonable time and has the option of doing several things. For example, the trainer (1) might ask for a show of hands on each item on the list or (2) use the list as a lead-in for a didactic presentation. There are various ways to handle the icebreaker, but the important point is that its primary uses are as a tension reliever, to build an esprit de corps, and to encourage quick participation in the learning experience.

Quarterly Core Programs

Acute care facilities and SNFs tend to have high personnel turnover rates. For many SNFs, and particularly those in urban communities, personnel changes

Figure 5–3 Example of Slide Used in Generic Disaster Training

Purposes of Emergency Preparedness

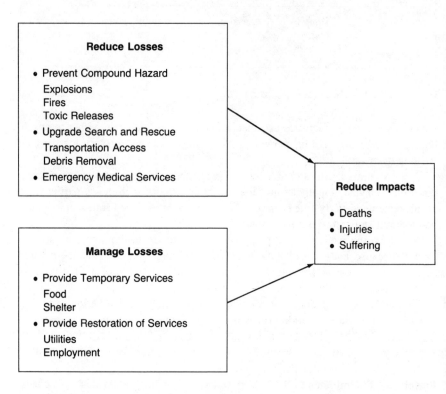

Source: Reprinted with permission of the California Governor's Earthquake Task Force, 1982.

exceeding 200 percent annually are not uncommon. While generally more stable, acute care facilities also have their difficulties with turnover. The growing reliance on contract, temporary, and part-time personnel and outside vendors has produced a situation in which a facility may be staffed continually by large numbers of "new" people. The widespread practice of handing new employees the *Disaster Manual* to read, or holding a brief program on the subject during their first week on the job, does not and will not prepare them adequately.

Quarterly core programs are the best mechanism for training new employees. Although as long as three months may pass before some new staff members have participated in these programs, systematic training is a requisite if all personnel are expected to respond appropriately to a disaster.

Exhibit 5–8 Example of an "Icebreaker" Handout

Myths and Realities About Disasters		
Please check whether you agree or disagree:	*Agree*	*Disagree*

1. Most people panic in a disaster situation.
2. A hospital's emergency care system and its disaster emergency care system actually are two ends of the same continuum.
3. One element that prevents health care organizations from working together is conflicting regulations.
4. Planning assumes that it is really possible to control the future.
5. The greatest barrier to effective disaster planning is lack of money.
6. Small hospitals would be safer places to be than large hospitals in a nuclear attack on our community.
7. Disaster situations "create" natural leaders.
8. Clinical personnel are more dependable in a disaster than are housekeeping personnel.
9. Most people are selfish and look out only for themselves in a disaster.
10. The greatest danger from an earthquake is falling into openings or fissures in the earth.
11. The triage assignment in a disaster raises ethical issues.
12. People act alike in a disaster—there is no difference between men and women, old and young, etc.

Training-of-Trainers Programs

Facilitywide disaster preparedness training is time consuming. Training others to carry out aspects of the training can be of considerable help in reaching everyone in the institution.

Specialized training will be necessary if managers, supervisors, or personnel other than the Disaster Coordinator are expected to conduct follow-up training (see below). Training trainers is an excellent way to spread knowledge and to motivate management. Any training-of-trainers program should include the following:

- in-depth review of *Disaster Manual* specifications for the various departments
- expanded training in the psychology of disaster preparedness
- instruction in training methods for teaching adult learners and evaluating learning.

If trainers are expected to maintain class attendance rosters, develop course materials, and evaluate behavioral changes after the presentation, they must be shown how to fulfill these responsibilities.

Follow-Up Training Programs

Follow-up training should take place as soon as possible after the core program. Such scheduling establishes the seriousness of disaster preparedness and provides for the expansion of individual knowledge and skills. Too often, facility training programs lose momentum after a strong initial program.

For example, one large urban hospital spent a great deal of money to provide 400 employees with an all-day "disaster retreat" workshop at a convention center. Experts from government, local universities, and consulting firms spoke and responded to questions. People seemed to enjoy the day immensely and discussed the benefits of the program when they returned to work. However, nothing happened for almost a year. Instead, department heads were sent a copy of the facility manual and asked to circulate it among their staffs. The excitement generated by the workshop faded and the manuals were shelved quickly.

Two types of follow-up programs are helpful: department/work unit programs and drills. Examples of each are detailed next.

DEPARTMENT/WORK UNIT TRAINING PROGRAMS

Subelement Classes

These classes can be scheduled in 30-minute or one-hour time frames. Their purpose is to present information on single elements of the *Disaster Manual* so that all staff members become familiar with how each subelement of the manual works. Subelements include personnel notification procedures, location and procurement of equipment and supplies, Triage Area activities, evacuation procedures, use of paperwork, etc. The material provided should be specific and appropriate for each individual area mobilized during a disaster.

Subelement classes may be held monthly, rotating departments/work units for each presentation. Department managers and unit supervisors can be trained to provide the content as part of their normal responsibility for employee training and development. Exhibit 5–9 and Exhibit 5–10 are examples of subelement class outlines.

Plan Review at Unit Staff Meetings

Staff meetings are a good forum for a quick, informal review (five to ten minutes) of unit disaster responses and responsibilities. Topics can include loca-

Exhibit 5–9 Example of Outline for Subelement Class: Staff Recall

Outline

1. Brief review of overall notification system
2. Review of staff recall work sheet
3. Location of confidential recall work sheet on the unit
4. Who will make the decision to recall, and when
5. Who will be assigned recall
6. Documentation on the work sheet
7. What to do when called to respond while off duty
8. Paper flow of work sheet when documentation is complete
9. Questions/answers

tion and use of the unit manual, public address system announcements for disaster alert, location and mobilization of unit disaster-related equipment and supplies, and decision-making criteria for unit response. The fact that the supervisor takes the time to include brief reviews of the practical aspects is positive reinforcement for the philosophy that disaster preparedness is a continual process.

Spot Review on the Job

Another useful technique for supervisors and the Disaster Coordinator while on daily rounds is to stop and informally ask questions of personnel: "What would you do right now if a disaster alert were announced?" or "How would you initiate patient evacuation from your unit if this wing was damaged in an earthquake?" These can provide a wealth of information regarding readiness and future training needs as well as the impact of past training.

Exhibit 5–10 Example of Outline for Subelement Class: Immediate Response to a Facility Fire

Outline

1. Definition of an "internal" disaster
2. What to do immediately if you find a fire
3. What to do immediately if you hear the fire bell
4. Procedure for securing the area
5. Protecting yourself
6. Procedures for evacuating patients
7. Questions/answers

DRILLS

Simulated disaster experiences can build effectively upon core program training and follow-ups. Disaster plans are only theories of performance. Many of those for whom the plan is developed have minimal awareness of how all of its parts and roles dovetail. Experience in simulations provides the opportunity to perform in a controlled environment. While essential for hands-on practice and decision making, drills should not take place until participants have attended the core program and follow-up subelement classes.

Simulation drills are quite helpful in:

- enabling individuals to integrate current skills with new ones
- providing a forum for evaluating plan effectiveness, efficiency, and feasibility
- setting the stage for testing new ideas and methods
- testing procedures, decision–making processes, and criteria for judgment
- promoting intrafacility and interfacility cooperation and coordination
- providing a forum for review and critique of the existing plan.

The Joint Commission on Accreditation of Hospitals (JCAH) requires that acute care facilities conduct two exercises annually.[1] The types of simulation presented here, and mock-casualty exercises discussed in this chapter, all provide a means for qualitative evaluation of the disaster plan and provide similar outcomes. If these are documented fully, requirements for the JCAH will be met.

Disaster drills are not a panacea, althouth many view them as such. There are myths about drills that are not correct. Disaster drills do not:

- ensure compliance with the disaster plan
- have to be a surprise to be valid
- have to include mock casualties and be comprehensive to be valid
- test only performance—they also can educate.

Planners interested in using drill experiences as learning tools should consider the following in developing them:

What Type of Drill Will Be Most Appropriate?

This decision involves such variables as the frequency and success of prior disaster drills, personnel turnover and training schedules, and accreditation and regulatory requirements. It takes significantly longer to plan for and implement a major mock-casualty exercise involving many other resources than it takes, for example, to hold a paper or tabletop drill.

What Is the Goal of the Drill?

To paraphrase Goethe: "Before you can know where you are going, you must know where you want to be." As Disaster Planning Committee members begin discussing the elements of a drill, they may find their deliberations skewed by outside pressures. There are times when facilities become involved in a major mock-casualty drill because an outside agency decides to have one and invites area health care facilities to participate. The decision to go ahead should be based primarily on the institution's own training needs and not on another organization's priorities.

What Are the Drill Objectives?

These should state clearly what is to be tested and accomplished. For example: "The April 27 drill will test the *response times* of the following units: Triage Area, Command Post, Personnel Pool, Inhouse transportation services, and Major Treatment Area." The objectives establish a framework for defining tasks and time frames, developing the drill, and evaluating effectiveness (see Exhibit 5–11).

Who Will Be Involved in Planning?

The institution's Disaster Planning Committee usually is the primary group involved in the planning and scheduling of intrafacility drills. However, experts from elsewhere in the facility and from the community should be involved as appropriate. It is important to identify resource persons early in the planning and involve them throughout drill development to avoid critical oversights. It can be extremely disconcerting to be in the middle of a major exercise and find that vital resources never were included in the planning. Many times this one oversight may cause a drill to be of little or no real value.

Utilizing outside resources in planning drills enhances cooperation in real events. For example, one chronic care facility involved the National Guard in its drill-planning processes. The scenario assumed that a flood disrupted the auxillary power in the facility. The Guard was to deliver and set up mobile generators, and some essential services in the facility were to be suspended while this was being done. The irony was that while drill planning was in progress, the facility actually experienced the exact scenario: the basement flooded when a nearby irrigation channel overflowed. As in the planned scenario, the National Guard was called to bring mobile generators to take over essential disrupted services. The closeness of reality and drill planning certainly revealed the need for including community resources in facility disaster response drills.

Exhibit 5–11 Example of Work Sheet for Developing Objectives

Objective Work Sheet

(Check all applicable areas)

A. *Format*

The objective is to: Test _____ Train _____ Both _____

The exercise should be: Announced _____ Unannounced _____

B. *Scope of Involvement*

	Will Be Tested	Will Not Be Tested
Sorting at Scene		
First Aid at Scene		
Transportation		
Sorting at Hospitals		
Identification/Records		
External Communications		
Internal Communications		
Supplies		
Utilization of Services		
Emergency Dept.		
Surgery		
X-ray		
Laboratory		
Patient Floors		
Other _____		

C. *Level of Personnel Involvement*

	Mgmt. Only	Mgmt. & Staff	None
Administration			
Medical Staff			
Emergency Dept.			
Surgery			
X-ray			
Laboratory			
Central Service			
Maintenance/Engineering			
Purchasing/Supplies			
Security			
Nursing Floors			
Dietary			
Pharmacy			
Medical Records			
Other _____			

D. *Outside Participation of Related Agencies*

	Active	Observations	None
Ambulance Companies			
American Red Cross			
Civil Defense			
Fire Department			
Medical Association			
Law Enforcement			
Specify _____			
Other _____			

Source: Adapted from *Assessing Your Hospital's Disaster Plan and Disaster Drills,* Hospital Council of Southern California, Office of Professional Services, 1983.

Large-scale interfacility drills generally are coordinated by a Multiagency Disaster Drill Planning Committee. Each participating facility should be represented. Even if such a committee has overall responsibility, the facility's own Disaster Planning Committee should be actively preparing for the facility's own response.

Who Will Be Involved in the Drill?

Drills are practice events that affect the work and personal lives of employees at all levels and often affect inhouse patients and community citizens as well. The "people" aspects of drill planning must be considered carefully. Only those who because of their roles are integral to the drill should be involved. Otherwise, essential facility services may be disrupted unnecessarily, fiscal costs of the exercise will escalate, and considerable patient and personnel resentment may be generated. Those who are to be involved should be informed of the drill and the approximate or specific date and time, except in the infrequent instance of a "surprise" mock-casualty drill.

What Will Be the Scenario?

Planners must attempt to establish a realistic drill scenario. The range of choices is enormous—ideas are as close as the headlines of the newspaper or articles in emergency care publications such as *Emergency Medical Services* and the *Journal of Emergency Nursing*. The Disaster Planning Committee might consider several possible scenarios, basing its selection on the following criteria:

- Is it likely to be instructive?
- Will it motivate participants?
- Is it realistic to this facility and locale?

Following is a partial list of possible scenarios:

- bus accident with multiple victims
- train derailment
- chemical spill
- medical nuclear isotope spill
- aircraft accident
- terrorist activity at a sporting event
- gas explosion in an industrial plant
- bomb explosion in the facility
- riot during a rock concert at the local entertainment center
- fire in a downtown convention hotel

The scenario sets the scale of the event and suggests the type of personnel and community resources that must be involved in the planning. If the drill does not involve facility–community agency collaboration, outside community resources will not have to be identified. However, expert public safety personnel still should be consulted.

What Time and Date Shall the Drill Be Held?

The time should complement the objectives. Mock-casualty drills should be held at realistic times; for instance, a tornado is an unlikely midwinter event in the northeastern states. A drill involving earthquake victims would be more effective if a "worst case" scenario is established, meaning that, for example, the drill is held during traffic rush hour when victims would be generated from workplaces, residences, and roadways. Tabletop drills, paper drills, and board games can be developed as alternatives to such exercises. Their time and date should be established to involve as many staff members as possible, but also to include other shifts. Therefore, such drills also should be held during shifts other than the day shift with an appropriate scenario—regardless of drill type.

Surprise should not be the purpose of a drill. If people are caught seemingly unprepared, either they lack the training to respond effectively or the plan requires an unworkable response. In disaster preparedness training, the axiom should be: No surprises until all personnel are trained thoroughly and the plan is carefully tested.

Who Will Evaluate the Outcome?

Drill auditors should be recruited to observe and document behavioral responses specified by training program objectives. In some cases, auditors also must be able to instruct and coach.

Auditors can be drawn from the Disaster Planning Committee membership, although experienced and knowledgeable individuals from other facilities and/or agencies also can be recruited. Whoever acts as auditor must be well versed in the facility plan, the goals and objectives of the drill, the anticipated outcomes, and the use of scoring forms.

What Are the Criteria for a Successful Outcome?

The Disaster Planning Committee should determine effectiveness criteria for all major exercises. If there is no facility Disaster Coordinator, the committee would also have to develop outcome criteria for lesser scale simulations such as paper drills. These criteria are essential for retrospective and progressive auditing of the drill and must be measurable. Table 5–4 is an example of a drill critique form for retrospective audit. The form specifies action indicators, their referencing in the manual, the determined standard, and acceptable exceptions from the standard.

Table 5–4 Example of a Retrospective Disaster Audit Form

Element	Where Found	Standard 100%	Exception	Comments
Times:				
1. Call received by HEAR operator	HEAR* log, situation report	Within 1 minute		
2. HEAR operator responds	HEAR log	Within 1 minute		
3. Administration notified	Emergency situation report	Within 2 minutes		
4. Nursing office notified	Emergency situation report	Within 3 minutes		
5. Emergency Administration notified	Emergency situation report			
6. First Staff call—Emergency Department	Staff phone roster	Within 5 minutes	Fewer than 5 disaster patients	
7. ED Command Center open	Initial notification form	Within 5 minutes	Fewer than 10 disaster patients	
8. Triage Area established	ED Command Center log	Within 5 minutes	Fewer than 5 disaster patients	
9. Auxiliary Departments notified: X-ray, Lab, Housekeeping, Engineering, Central Service, Surgery, Recovery, IV Team	ED Command Center log	Within 5 minutes	X-ray, Lab only notified if more than 10 patients; Surgery notified if more than 5 patients to be received	
10. Special care areas notified: ICU, CCU, Surgical ICU	Administration disaster log	Within 5 minutes	Fewer than 5 patients to be received	

*HEAR = Hospital Emergency Administrative Radio

When Will Critique Sessions Be Held?

If at all possible, individual work units should hold informal follow-up critique sessions immediately after drills are completed. A formal follow-up critique usually is held several days later and involves all of the participants in the drill. (The critique session concept is discussed later in this chapter.)

Types of Drills

These can include any or all of the following: simulation board games, paper drills, tabletop drills, subsystem drills, and mock casualty exercise.

Simulation Board Games

Disaster manuals, training programs, and even major drill exercises do not provide enough contingencies to simulate the complexity of a real event. In reality, unanticipated contingencies are the norm. Board games provide a remedy for this problem. Most people have had some prior experience with the game Monopoly, for instance, and are comfortable with a game format and with competition among players. A disaster board game can be fun and educational at the same time. The following is a description of a board game devised by the management development coordinator of an acute care hospital.

Game players are asked to respond to a hypothetical disaster. Because this hospital virtually straddles the San Andreas Fault, the game postulates a major earthquake scenario. Players are assigned the roles specified in the manual. The game operator acts as scorekeeper and casts the dice to determine the month the disaster strikes. A dial is spun to determine day of week and time. Location cards tell the players where they are when the disaster strikes. Chance cards pose contingencies and consequences that players have to respond to.

When a player (or team of players) makes a decision, dice are tossed and/or a wheel is spun to add variables to the situation mix. Winners can be determined by any number of criteria, including total points earned (for the right responses) and correctness of decision making and judgment.

This type of game is a creative way to acquire information and encourage flexibility and risk taking in decisions. Other types of games that might be developed include "Disaster Jeopardy" and "Disaster Trivial Pursuit." The possibilities are endless, limited only by imagination. Anything that stimulates critical thinking, decision making, and debate will enhance learning.

Paper Drills

Paper drills are an excellent tool for evaluating behavior in a controlled setting, and to evaluate thought processes in subelement testing. In this type of drill a disaster is announced and participants are expected to complete all appropriate paper work, make telephone notifications, etc., that relate to the scenario. For example, one facility wanted to test its ability to evacuate patients. While no one actually was moved, all proper notifications and paper work were completed just as they would be in a real situation. The only element missing is the actual receipt of casualties and/or the actual movement of patients. Exhibit 5–12 is an example of a form used to document simulated patient movement in a countywide disaster drill.

Tabletop Drills

The tabletop drill is performed in a classroom setting and involves management and/or staff members from appropriate departments. After a scenario is presented, participants are asked to respond to a series of problems written on 3″ × 5″ cards and placed in individual envelopes. The methodology of the drill is as follows:

- Participants are assembled in a conference-style setting and grouped by department, i.e., Radiology, Emergency Services, Housekeeping, Medical Records, etc. Trainers might ask each group to identify itself with a large, colored placard.
- A prior planned time frame and scenario is given to the participants (usually one to one and a half hours).
- Audiovisual aids simulate the scenario as it unfolds. For example, a tape recording of the initial facility notification can help provide aural realism and videos and slides visual realism.
- While one trainer manages the process, two or three proctors in the room guide the flow, handing out problem envelopes at strategic moments, and observing and documenting responses.
- The drill begins as it would in actuality. Departments that are expected to respond first in an actual event are asked to state what they will do when they are first notified.
- Problem (contingency) cards inside sealed envelopes are handed out at intervals. Some cards are blank, and the departments receiving these will have to determine for themselves what is happening at that moment and what possible problems they might be facing. Contingencies may range from "There has been a fire from broken gas lines in the laundry room" to "The basement has flooded." To heighten realism and excitement, trainers can make up additional contingencies as the drill unfolds.
- Patient cards identifying arriving casualties are used to determine casualty flow from Triage to designated receiving units. The cards can be laid out on a

Exhibit 5–12 Example of Paper Drill Element

Patient Simulated Movement Form*

Name of Patient _____ Room # _____
Diagnosis _____
Doctor _____
        (Enter patient's initials, diagnosis, and doctor on the form. You are to use actual
        patients on the units.)

1. Discharge Assessment at _____ A.M./P.M. by _____
    (Enter whatever time you begin this phase of your plan.)

2. Attending Physician Called at _____ A.M./P.M. by _____
    (If your facility delegates this authority to the house physician, indicate this.)

3. Attending Physician Responded
    (This is the time that the physician responded to your call. If house physicians, it
    will be the time they came to the unit.)
    Discharge: Yes ( )   No ( )

4. Family Called at _____ A.M./P.M. by _____

5. Family Responded Yes ( ) at _____ A.M./P.M.   No ( ) A.M./P.M.
    Will Pick Up Patient at _____ A.M./P.M.
    (Answers to 4 and 5 will be estimates unless you have decided to involve the
    families.)

6. Patient Dressed & Ready at _____A.M./P.M.
    (Estimate how long you think it would take for this particular patient to be dressed
    and ready.)

7. Patient Taken to Business Office at _____ A.M./P.M. by _____
    Amb. ( )   Stretcher ( )   W/C ( )
    Business Office Transaction Completed at _____ A.M./P.M.
    Please have Business Office date, time, and initial this section.)

8. Patient Taken to Holding Area _____ A.M./P.M. by _____
    (Have someone in the Holding Area initial this section.)

or

9. Patient Left Hospital at _____ A.M./P.M.
    (#8 or #9 will be estimated times.)

10. Room Cleaned & Ready at _____ A.M./P.M.

  *The Patient Simulated Movement Form is designed to assist you in estimating the actual
time it will take to discharge patients in the event of a major emergency.

Source: Reprinted with permission from Sadonya Antebe, Los Angeles County Department of Health Services, Disaster
Services.

---

table for easier manipulation by Triage Area personnel. When a casualty moves from Triage to a receiving area, the patient card is given to the appropriate participants, who then must state what they will do with the victim. Time lags are normal during a disaster and should be provided for in the drill to maximize realism. (Participants should be polled during time lags to identify what they believe they would be doing during an actual time lag.)

- When a department performs a procedure involving another department, the latter is the next to respond to a problem card. For example, if the ED reports it has received notification of a disaster and that, according to plan, it is notifying PBX, a proctor hands the notification card to PBX, which then states what it will do.

- Work sheets developed in advance are given to all participants to involve them in the drill. These are simple forms with lines, date, department, and name of responder. They are used by every participant to write observations, questions, suggestions, problems, ideas, and thoughts as they occur. The work sheets are collected by the proctors at the end of the program and reviewed later.

Tabletop drills can be as elaborate as the coordinator wants them to be. However, they still are significantly less expensive than an exercise utilizing mock casualties. There are many benefits to tabletop drills:

- They provide a controlled setting in which to guide participants through a disaster response.

- Responses to scenario development can be evaluated much more easily than in a mock-patient drill, which tends to get out of control very easily.

- The major elements they test are disaster management principles and problem solving, but the process is much less threatening than a mock-patient drill because it is in a closed setting.

- All plan elements and subelements can be tested. In fact, the tabletop drill is a good test for the newly revised plan after personnel have been taught the revisions.

- Elements of the disaster plan that traditionally are problems in actual disaster response can be evaluated more carefully. For example, inadequate intra-organizational and interorganizational communications are common in disasters because of information overload (or inadequacies), confused and distorted messages, and absence of trained communication personnel. These elements can be tested and evaluated during a tabletop drill and the necessary judgment to respond to these contingencies can be developed in the controlled setting.

- Individuals can be allowed to work spontaneously, thinking up contingencies themselves or making suggestions to other departments about possible actions.

The elements needed to stage a successful tabletop drill include:

- a written statement of purpose for all participants
- a written rationale for disaster preparedness, including definition of disaster
- audiovisual aids as appropriate:

slides
transparencies
problem cards
sealed envelopes with unplanned problems
work sheets
two-way radios
blackboard
critique forms

Subsystem Drills

Subsystem drills are designed to test and evaluate specific sections of the *Disaster Manual*, such as Command Post operations, Communications, Triage Area operations, paper work, etc.

Any element of the plan can be selected for testing. This type of drill most appropriately follows in sequence from didactic training to paper, tabletop, and then to subsystem drills. Subsystem drills should not be held until personnel are familiar with disaster response patterns in the facility.

Steps to follow for planning and implementing a subsystem drill include the following:

Select an Element To Test. It is best to concentrate initially on only one element at a time. Over time, several elements can be mixed to test more than one aspect of the plan in anticipation of a large-scale mock-victim drill. It is advisable, however, to start small and expand as knowledge grows, as training is accomplished, and as the plan demonstrates its integrity in single element testing.

Establish a Scenario. The scenario should be realistic and scaled appropriate to the element being evaluated.

Define Drill Objectives. The next step is to determine which aspects of the element will be tested. An example of element testing is the paper work drill. Objectives of a paper work drill can include: (1) locating work sheets, tags, action cards, etc., (2) identifying persons responsible for completing paper work and the circumstances for doing so, and (3) identifying and improving the flow of paper work. If the Command Post operation is to be evaluated, for example, objectives might be to clarify personnel roles and reporting relationships and to test the priorities of equipment and supply allocations. If response time is the only factor to be evaluated, personnel should be advised in advance and performance objectives should be reviewed at that time. In this subelement drill, coaching onsite is inadvisable because that will prolong response times and skew results.

Mock-Casualty Exercises

As mentioned earlier, large-scale, interfacility/agency drills generally are managed by a Multiagency Disaster Drill Planning Committee.* This committee's role is to coordinate, reduce duplication, and maximize resources. Membership in it is a must if a facility intends to take an active role in a multiagency mock-casualty exercise. Participating in a large-scale drill involving many areas of the institution, other facilities, and field care providers is a major undertaking. It is a dress rehearsal for the real thing. Because of its scale, the mock-casualty drill may not be cost or learning effective unless personnel have already been thoroughly trained in manual use and disaster response concepts. The reality is that many facilities are unprepared to structure, participate in, or manage a mock-casualty exercise and should consider participating in a large-scale drill carefully.

Questions to consider before becoming involved are:

- Has the institution clearly defined its own goal and objectives for the drill? Each facility should identify specific areas it wishes to test in its own organization and determine whether these needs can be met by the multi-agency drill. Facilities in the process of training personnel in disaster preparedness, those in the plan revision stage, and those who have not yet completed their own smaller scale drills are not in the best position to benefit much from the large-scale mock-casualty drill.

- Are the plan and manual in a state of readiness appropriate to facilitywide testing? If not, it may be better to initiate the other training and testing activities suggested earlier before taking the time and allocating the resources for a major drill. Such a drill involves so much more planning, players, and process that to participate in one simply because it seems like a good idea would be counterproductive and costly. Although community agencies may plan multiorganizational drills, the decision to collaborate should be weighed against the facility's own level of preparedness.

---

*Multiagency committees are created by public safety agencies in some communities, by County Disaster Services Coordinators in others, or by hospitals in a community seeking to collaborate.

- Is the institution ready to stage receipt of mock casualties and to critique its operation? All forms, equipment, and process audits should be ready if the benefits of a mock exercise on a facilitywide and/or communitywide basis are to be realized. The facility must be in such a state of readiness that it is able to concentrate on interfacility and interagency teamwork, cooperation, and comprehensive planning, and to evaluate the overall disaster operation through a well-developed critique and audit process. The most important single factor in the success of a multifacility and agency disaster exercise is effective organization of the participants.[2]

The critical factor in the success of facility response to such a drill is a plan that has been tested already during inhouse drills and personnel who have been well trained in all aspects of the facility plan and manual. In the absence of this, the exercise may be futile and, at worst, hinder preparedness.

If and when facility disaster planners decide to go ahead with a large-scale exercise, planning efforts must be coordinated with area facilities and agencies. The appropriate vehicle for doing so is the community's Multiagency Disaster Drill Planning Committee or its equivalent. Large-scale exercises require extensive discussion and consensus regarding the following factors.

Drill Objectives

Several factors should be considered:

- whether the drill should be announced publicly via the media
- the drill objectives of each collaborating facility and agency
- the levels of personnel from each facility who will be involved
- the expectations of the planners.

The sample work sheet shown in Exhibit 5–11 (above) can be used in preparing objectives for a collaborative drill.

Disaster Event Scenario

The scenario is a vital element upon which all planning activities and drill response patterns are based. The scenario defines the magnitude of the event and should be developed with geographical, socioeconomic, and community health and planning needs in mind. Selection of scenarios should vary with each exercise so that different aspects of system response can be tested at different times.

Victim Scenario

How many victims, what type of injuries, and what type of victim role training and makeup will be required must be determined. Victim volunteers can be recruited from many sources but it is best to select those with some medical background so that role programming is maintained. Student nurses, residents and interns, college premed students, and Boy Scouts and Girl Scouts all are valuable resources, as will be discussed later.

Selecting a Date for the Exercise

Numerous factors are involved in selecting the date and time for a large-scale drill. The availability of victims, physicians, nurses, public safety resources, and volunteers (who are needed for a variety of jobs, including makeup), staging areas near the disaster site, and transportation resources all will affect the scheduled drill date. The Multiagency Disaster Drill Planning Committee should assess each of these factors against the need for a realistic time to run the scenario. A lead time of at least four months is recommended for scheduled events.[3]

Involving Community Agencies

If a facility is initiating the drill, its Disaster Planning Committee must determine the point at which agencies such as police, fire, private ambulance companies, service clubs, the Red Cross, and community disaster preparedness planners should become involved. It is best for the committee that intiates the drill to maintain control of planning and coordination of operations.[4] Local planners from state disaster and/or emergency agencies also should be included in drill planning meetings.

Selecting a Disaster Site

The site should be realistic. If an industrial explosion is to be simulated, the site should be in or near an industrial area. Planners should select a site that meets these criteria: (a) it has no recognized hazards, (b) it is near the staging site where "victims" can be prepared and from which transportation can be dispatched, and (c) it is securable. Law enforcement, Chambers of Commerce, Red Cross, and other agencies can be helpful in selecting and/or ensuring the availability of a particular site.

Transportation

Arrangements will have to be made for the movement of volunteer victims from the staging site to the disaster site, from the disaster site to receiving facilities, and from the receiving facilities back to staging at the end of the exercise. Because there is some inherent danger in rescue vehicle operations during a drill, decisions will have to be made as to what routes the rescue vehicles will travel when responding and retrieving victims, whether lights and sirens will be used, and what will be done if normal, daily emergencies occur elsewhere during the drill.[5]

Public safety agencies often arrange for standby equipment and personnel to meet normal EMSS needs during the drills. In areas where it is difficult to do this, specific arrangements will have to be made so that all units are not deployed to the mock disaster, leaving the community unprotected by rescue personnel. Onsite public safety command personnel will manage unexpected problems involving rescue vehicle deployment, traffic patterns, and victim loading. These persons also should be prepared to alter the scenario if abrupt changes occur in the weather.

All transportation agencies will appreciate receiving written verification, at least two weeks before the drill, of travel routes to and from the disaster site, and selected ground rules for use of vehicle lights, sirens, and speed. Discussion and input from prehospital (paramedic) provider agencies should be sought during the planning process. If helicopter services are to be used, their operators must be included in the planning. Participants must be advised if they are expected to use private cars for any purpose other than their own transportation to and from the staging area.

Selecting the Staging Area

Selection of the staging area depends on availability and approximation to the disaster site. The site should be large enough to allow for the following:

- parking for all volunteer private autos
- staging for all rescue vehicles (including turnaround areas)
- makeup and moulage areas (preferably sheltered from the weather)
- holding of casualties for deployment to the disaster site
- canteen for meals and/or refreshments
- registration of participants
- sanitary facilities
- fencing
- proximity to participating hospitals and to the disaster site.

Cover protection for participants in the event the weather changes should be anticipated and planned for. Because a great deal of equipment, supplies, and personal belongings will remain in the staging area, the plan must provide security as well. If the media are involved, the press should be assigned to a separate area and allowed controlled entrance during the time makeup and moulage take place. The best strategy is not to allow anyone other than specifically authorized and identified participants into the staging area.

Disaster Site and Staging Area Coordinators

Both the disaster site and staging area must be managed. The most appropriate coordinator or manager for the disaster site is a fire commander experienced in the performance of a disaster drill. The staging area can be coordinated by a health facility administrator experienced in disaster drills. Assigned coordinators should be the highest-ranking authority in each area. The Staging Area Coordinator also is responsible for the return of the site to its original condition and the return of equipment and supplies.

Sequence of Events

The format for drill sequence must be worked out well in advance of the event. If it is not, vital notifications can be overlooked and participants in the drill (particularly those who have been planning to receive victims) may not benefit adequately from the experience. Communication is crucial: who initiates the drill, dispatches transportation, and alerts the facilities should be predetermined. Once the sequence of events has been developed, a checklist can be made to enable progressive evaluation of events by proctors. This information then can be used during the formal critique session following the drill.

Public Information Program

Public information and security issues must be addressed well in advance of the drill date. If the public is to be aware of the exercise and/or be involved, a public information program must be developed. The Multiagency Disaster Drill Planning Committee can develop and distribute news releases itself or it may depend upon individual facilities to do so. Media relations are very important. TV pictures and newspaper accounts can be helpful both in preparing for the drill and in publicizing its outcomes. The local media tend to be interested in mock drills. Many institutions have been able to involve stations in the production of related TV and radio programming that teaches citizens about survival strategies and their role in preparedness.

All public announcements must be prefaced by the words "THIS IS A DRILL." Photographers from the media usually want to be at the site. Their presence often lends an air of realism to the event. To limit confusion, all media at the staging or drill sites should be asked to wear an identifiable symbol. Some TV crews wear large bibs with station name and call letters for identification purposes.

Drill Preannouncement

Information should be developed for distribution to participating public safety agencies and health facilities. Most drills of this magnitude cannot be maintained for long as a "surprise." Word always leaks out. However, as noted earlier, surprise drills generally are not beneficial, nor do they tend to meet their stated objectives. Personnel should be encouraged to begin their own preparation by reviewing their institution's disaster plan and manual. Correct response activities are reinforced more by a drill that proceeds smoothly and correctly than one that falters and has many errors.[6]

Participating facilities and agencies can announce the month in which the drill will be held without revealing details; the nature of the event (scenario particulars) also can be kept confidential if appropriate.

"Victims" Readiness

As the time for the drill approaches, several tasks must be carried out to prepare casualty resources. Recruiting of "victims" should begin no less than one month before the event. There are likely to be some volunteers from the health facilities although, if possible, those individuals should be retained for the operating response. Many facilities use their nonpaid volunteers as victims. The drawback here is that these persons often are well known to staff members and, on occasion, more chatting and socializing occurs than is desirable. In addition, volunteers often lack sufficient background in medical care and do not retain victim role programming as well. On the other hand, their "layperson behavior" often is realistic. If facility lay volunteers are enlisted, or if any others with limited or no medical background are used, careful and methodical scripting of injuries and responses will be necessary. Finally, the victim actors selected should approximate the age range of the victims in the scenario. For example, a school bus accident requires school-age children as victims, an industrial plant explosion calls for more male victims, and so forth.

If children are to be used, prior parental consent must be obtained for use of the minor both as a victim and for medical treatment should an unforseen injury or illness occur during the drill. In addition, children have special needs that must be taken into account, such as the need for frequent snacks and fluids, accessible sanitary facilities, and protection from weather and equipment hazards.

All victims must be assembled in a meeting before the event to provide them with an orientation, a profile of the sequence of activities, and details such as meal arrangements, parking, the names and phone numbers of coordinators, and the exact date and time that they are to assemble at the staging area. Exhibit 5–13 outlines the information that should be given during the orientation.

Programming of victim injuries and behavior should begin at this meeting. All victims must be coached carefully to understand their injuries and respond accordingly. They also should be given an information card that notes their injuries and condition, the makeup that will be required and applied in the staging area, and responses congruent with injuries that will be needed by field triagers and ED personnel in order to perform triage correctly. The actors then can study this

Exhibit 5–13 Example of Participant Instruction Sheet

WELCOME!

Thank you for helping us.

The hospitals and your community are conducting a simulated emergency drill to test their ability to respond to a genuine catastrophe, should one occur in this area.

Your participation in this exercise is an extremely important factor in helping us to learn. Without your help, this project would be meaningless. We value your assistance and are grateful to you for volunteering your free time.

Exercise Details:

Date _____ Report to Staging Area at _____A.M./P.M.
Approximate Duration: _____
Staging Area Location: _____
Participating Hospitals: _____ _____
_____ _____ _____

Arrangements: (Describe where applicable)

Parking:

Transportation:

Lunch:

Suggestions:

Be on time.

Wear old, old clothes. You may be a victim, which requires your clothes to be torn, cut, or burned. You may be required to lie on the ground.

For personal comfort and safety, wear full type low-heeled shoes.

Listen to general directions and to your group leader.

Be careful at all times.

Source: Adapted from *Assessing Your Hospital's Disaster Plan and Disaster Drills*, Hospital Council of Southern California, Office of Professional Services, 1983.

---

information in advance of the drill. All victims requiring extensive moulage must be told to arrive early enough to be prepared properly for the drill. Others may arrive later. This may mean that two meals will have to be provided (breakfast/ lunch or lunch/dinner) during the event if victim preparation begins early. If the actors must complete Worker's Compensation and/or insurance forms, they should do so at the intial orientation meeting, not at the staging site on the day of the drill.

Programming victims (training them for their role) can be time consuming, depending on the extent and nature of their supposed injuries. Victim actors tend to comply with their role if the people who provide the orientation are serious and patient. At one drill critique, a mock victim was heard to say, "They told me I was supposed to be in shock, but no one told me what that was." Actors must be taught details of their injuries, how they occurred, and how they are supposed to behave. For training purposes, all terms must be defined specifically for participants. Knowledge of medical terms must not be taken for granted, even if student nurses or premed students are involved. The trainer should encourage feedback from victims. Any misinformation or misinterpretations should be corrected immediately. When the volunteers arrive at the staging area, their role may have to be reinforced once again.

Makeup and Moulage

This activity must be carefully planned because the realism of injuries and behavior is a decisive element for inhospital triage and emergency care. Moulage is a French term meaning a mold or cast made directly from and/or for a portion of the body and used to show a lesion or defect. The makeup and moulage are intended to make the mock victim appear to be injured, corresponding to the assigned role. For instance, if a nonpregnant woman is supposed to have complications of pregnancy compounded by injuries, her moulage would include giving her the appearance of a pregnancy. As described earlier, injuries are selected and assigned to victims in advance.

On the day of the drill, participants are made up and moulaged in the staging area. While trained makeup artists may be used, they are expensive; instead, volunteers can be trained to perform effective moulage. Emergency Medical Technician (EMT) course instructors usually have had some experience moulaging victims for training their own students and often are willing to assist in a disaster exercise. Many emergency nurses and EMTs have had such experience and may be willing to help out. A rule of thumb is to have one makeup person for each four victims. The more makeup people available the better because it generally takes 15 to 30 minutes to moulage a single victim, depending on the extent of injury. Because of this factor, volunteers should be scheduled to arrive at specific times for makeup; otherwise, they will have long, unnecessary waits.

Resources for material and moulage kits vary. Local Civil Defense offices, military bases, and EMT training programs may have materials available and may donate them. Commercial kits are expensive but include premade compounds that can be applied to body parts with spirit gum, an adhesive compound available at cosmetic stores and makeup artists supply stores. Adequate kits can be prepared by a moulage subcommittee of the Disaster Planning Committee.

The following are minimum supplies; all are commercially available and can be obtained in nontoxic form:

1. small plastic cups
2. small bowls
3. palette knives (available from artist stores, these are used to smooth wax and create lacerations in wax)
4. plastic squeeze bottles (used to hold solutions such as fake blood, glycerin, water, etc.)
5. tissues, tweezers, spray bottles, cotton balls
6. liquifying cleanser and cold cream (useful for removing makeup after the event or for correcting moulage mistakes during the makeup session; the cold cream is applied in a thin layer before makeup to make removal easier later)
7. soft foam makeup sponges (used to blend makeup for a realistic appearance)
8. several sizes of artist's brushes (#6-0)
9. alcohol or acetone (used to remove spirit gum, wax, and latex from body parts, excluding the eye area)
10. aeroplast spray (known commercially as "Fixit," the spray is a plastic sealer used to "set" moulaged wounds in place)
11. spirit gum
12. gelatin (useful for making third-degree burns)
13. Dermawax or Naturoplast: #1 firm (mortician's clay can be substituted for these commercially available products that are used to build up skin surface and blend fake bones into body parts)
14. petroleum jelly, cornstarch (petroleum jelly is used to make wounds appear "weepy," the cornstarch as powder to "set" makeup)
15. makeup: Clown white pancake makeup; blue shadow, yellow shadow, gray shadow; mortician's rouge or cream rouge (dark red); skin tone pancake in various shades; black pancake makeup; red, blue, yellow grease pencils; translucent powder and puffs (loose face powder)
16. maroon and crimson water colors, for simulated blood, available at most art stores (these paints also are available in tubes and can be used on abrasions and inside lacerations made in Dermawax to give an illusion of depth)
17. Karo syrup and red food coloring (used to make blood)
18. Duo surgical adhesive or liquid rubber latex (available at most drug stores or makeup stores, these substances are used to ensure adherence of molded materials to the skin)
19. instant oatmeal (mixed with water and appropriate food coloring, oatmeal can be held in the mouth and "vomited" at the appropriate moment)

20. "Crackel-it" (a substance for "aging" wood that can be found in hobby stores, this material can be used to make second-degree burns appear realistic)

The use of props will enhance the scenario. Anything realistic can be used. If wounds are to be dirty, grass or weeds can be placed into them or placed on hair and clothes. Old clothing should be worn by victims so it can be torn, burned, or made bloody during moulage.

Most injuries can be simulated with Dermawax and gelatin applied over spirit gum and/or latex. Simple conditions can be simulated, as follows:

Cyanosis: Place white pancake makeup, mixed with base colors and blue shadow, over earlobes, lips, around mouth, on the forehead, and on fingernails.

Diaphoresis: Use cotton balls to apply petroleum jelly over cold cream. Dilute the glycerin 1:1 with water and place in a spray bottle; spray over the petroleum jelly on forehead and upper lip (shield eyes, as glycerin makes them water).

Bruises: Rub red/blue shadow or grease sticks over bony prominences to simulate recent bruises; blue/yellow shadow or grease sticks simulate older bruises.

Abrasions: Dab brown/red/black grease sticks on area. Dapple blood over area with cotton balls. Use comb to gently scratch area in one direction. Dapple dirt over wound with cotton balls.

Black eyes: Apply red/blue rouge to depressions around eyes; do not connect the makeup at outside corner or the bruising will appear unrealistic.

Shock: Apply thin cold cream layer, then white pancake or grease stick over forehead and in creases around mouth. Use diaphoresis and cyanosis materials described above as appropriate. Apply a very thin layer of yellow/cream colored pancake or grease stick to forehead, cheekbones, and chin for a waxen appearance if profound shock is required. Paint area under the eyes and in cheek hollows with blue/gray grease sticks, then blend it with the yellow until the makeup appears realistic.

Blood: Simulate blood as either coagulated or uncoagulated. One formula for simulated blood is:

3 cups Karo syrup
10 teaspoons hot water
7 teaspoons red food coloring
1 teaspoon maroon water color
1 teaspoon crimson water color

To prevent "coagulation" add ⅛ teaspoon glycerin. If clots are desired, add equal parts of petroleum or KY jelly to red food coloring. Add blue food coloring drop by drop for effect.

Another formula, used by the Advanced Trauma Life Support training program, calls for combining and blending well the following ingredients (the amount of color is only approximate and is dependent upon the type and concentration of the food coloring used):

  1 pint white liquid starch
10 ml certified red food coloring
  3 ml certified yellow food coloring
  1 drop blue food coloring

Another type of simulated blood also is used by ATLS:

2 cups powdered sugar
1 teaspoon vanilla
1 fluid ounce certified red food coloring
1 teaspoon glycerin
1 cup dark Karo syrup (light Karo syrup may be used to achieve an arterial bleeding effect).[7]

To make a paste, combine and blend the first four ingredients well, then gradually add the rest of the ingredients to achieve the desired consistency. This blood has a sticky consistency—and has a pleasant taste.

Any of the blood solutions can be thinned as necessary by the addition of very small amounts of warm water.

Exhibits 5–14, 5–15, and 5–16 detail how to create three of the most common injuries: second- and third-degree burns and lacerations.

Successful wound simulation requires not only makeup but also realistic "staging" through the use of props and patient acting. Makeup artists must have a basic knowledge of the types of wounds to be simulated, good imagination, and the ingenuity necessary to create realistic simulations. As discussed earlier, victims should be aware of their signs and symptoms and be capable of portraying them in appropriate circumstances. They also must be coached carefully both at the orientation meeting and in the Staging Area on the day of the drill. If any changes in scenario or procedures have been instituted since their original indoctrination, reprogramming will be necessary.

Critique

During drill planning, the methodology for critiquing the event must be considered and developed. All progressive audit forms must be completed before the event, regardless of the type of drill being held. Examples of both progressive and retrospective audit evaluation forms appear earlier in this chapter. If nonfacility

Exhibit 5–14 Preparing Second–Degree Burn Makeup

---

red rouge
sponge
lip gloss, Duoplast, or Vaseline
tweezers
palette knife
Kleenex

1. apply rouge with foam sponge
2. apply Vaseline with knife, form into blisters, flatten some*
3. seal with Aeroplast, two or three applications
4. squeeze on Crackel-it, stipple and sponge (thin layer), dry well, stretch

   *Kryolan Tuplast produces good blisters; lip gloss also can be formed into blisters with a
palette knife and sealed with Aeroplast. Glycerin can be injected into a layer of Duo latex to
produce blisters.

---

observers participate in the audit process (for example, members of the Multi-agency Coordinating Disaster Exercise Planning Committee), it will be important to ensure that they use the same evaluation criteria when they are assessing facility response. Otherwise, it may be difficult to reconcile their observations with those made by facility-based observers.

Well in advance of the drill, observers must be trained in the use of progressive, retrospective, or combined audit forms. They need to know what to look for and what is expected of them. Exhibit 5–17 is an example of a critique planning guide to be used in assigning observers. Appendix 5–B presents a departmental critique checklist that can be used by an objective observer.

Two types of critique sessions are held after the drill: informal and formal. The names designate the process. An informal critique should be held immediately after a drill or actual disaster event is declared over. In this process the unit observer and/or manager gathers information from all participants, including victims, who were involved in their unit response. Observers ask the following questions:

- What do you think of the overall response to the drill event?
- What do you think went particularly well?
- What do you think needs improvement?
- Do you have any other suggestions and comments?

Questions should be kept brief and simple, with answers either put into writing or on a tape recorder for later transcription. Responses should be categorized

Exhibit 5–15 Preparing Third–Degree Burn Makeup

Gelatin
hot water
paper cup or bowl
spatula or end of brush
spirit gum
tweezers
Kleenex
red rouge
black makeup
rubber sponge
lip gloss or Vaseline

1. mix and make paste
2. apply to skin; as it sets, take knife and make surface irregular
3. spread latex or spirit gum over wound to seal
4. use sponge and stipple wound to keep gelatin from cracking
5. place one layer of Kleenex while latex is still wet
6. apply over area, tearing excess off
7. take tweezer, when dry, and lift areas of tissue off *especially from over gelatin* so skin looks raw
8. reseal with latex (the more sealed, the more it will stay)
9. let dry thoroughly (use hair dryer)
10. put dark red rouge on brush and paint indented areas where raw skin is
11. take sponge with black makeup and apply by stippling
12. make sure no white shows through
13. apply red around area; for areas of second-degree burns, apply at periphery
14. reapply red rouge so wound looks bloody
15. apply lip gloss to make wound look glossy
16. apply fresh blood in strategic areas

---

according to the classification of responder: i.e., physician, nurse, clerk, victim, etc. It is desirable to hold the informal critique with all of the participants in a unit assembled as a group. Patient needs and other requirements may preclude this, however. The alternative is individual interviews. Group interviews are preferred because (1) they take less time, (2) the group can brainstorm ideas, (3) one response often triggers recall in others, and (4) the group as a whole will be able to visualize what tasks lie ahead for correcting deficiencies in the plan.

If the group is gathered together for an informal critique as opposed to individual interviews, the meeting should be kept brief (just long enough for all to have the opportunity for input). If the meeting seems to require more time, another session can be set for problem solving, as long as the problem-sensing questions just listed are answered. This informal critique immediately after the event is essential for capturing reactions and sentiments before they are forgotten or

Exhibit 5–16 Preparing Laceration Makeup

---

spirit gum
Dermawax or Naturoplast
palette knife
Kleenex
Aeroplast
pan stick, Suntone
foam sponge
powder puff and loose powder
black makeup
red rouge
small brush
fake blood

1. apply thin layer of spirit gum under Naturoplast
2. spread thin layer of Naturoplast on skin
3. dot with Kleenex to make it look like skin
4. cut a laceration with palette knife, pull open slightly
5. spray Aeroplast and let dry
6. use foam sponge to dab Panstick over wound area
7. powder to take off shine
8. use small brush to dab Black Lightning into wound to add depth
9. dab red cream rouge into wound
10. fill laceration with fake blood

---

distorted. Because most formal critique sessions do not involve all participants, this may be the only time in which the experiences of many persons can be retrieved for subsequent review by the formal critique body.

A formal critique should be held no later than two weeks after the drill or real event has been declared over. The purpose of the interval is to allow time for unit managers to collect, evaluate, and collate progressive and retrospective audit data. Once that information is obtained, each manager identifies the strengths and weaknesses of the unit plan and of the facility plan and develops a report for the formal critique. Since recall tends to diminish rapidly, a formal critique held any later may not be as productive.

Regardless of how the formal critique is conducted, several elements are important to its success:

1. All of those expected to participate must be told, well in advance, of the meeting date and time.
2. The critique must be kept structured for the most efficient use of time. An agenda must be used and followed so that all areas and problems are presented. Minutes should be taken.

Exhibit 5–17 Critique Planning Guide

Date of Drill: _____

Type of critique observers are responsible for (circle one)
      Progressive   Retrospective   Both

Areas to be critiqued

   ___Triage   ___Command Post   ___Radiology
   ___Major Treatment   ___PBX   ___Surgery
   ___Delayed Care   ___Laboratory   ___Personnel Pool
   ___Security   ___Engineering

   Others: _____

Critique assignments:

Name	Location Assigned

---

3. The person chairing the meeting must have excellent group leadership skills and maintain control of the agenda.
4. Deficiencies in the Disaster Plan must be identified and prioritized.
5. Time frames for necessary revisions of plan or manual must be defined before the meeting is adjourned, and those responsible for action must be identified.
6. A date and location for the next meeting of the Disaster Planning Committee should be announced before the meeting adjourns.

CHANGING THE PLAN

Every drill and real disaster event is likely to uncover deficiencies in the disaster plan and manual because not every contingency for every type of event can be anticipated. A safe assumption is that drills and real events will result in either partial or total revision of the plan and manual. With each revision, retraining probably will be necessary, reflecting the axiom that disaster preparedness is a continuing process.

Problems must be evaluated carefully, plan revisions should take place according to a timetable, and written changes in the plan or manual should be distributed as soon as possible. Otherwise, another drill or real event may occur before the changes have been incorporated. Unfortunately, many facilities fall into this trap: they identify problems but do not adopt a systematic approach to resolving them. In time, the problems are forgotten and, when the next disaster incident or drill occurs, nothing has changed. The recycling of an ineffectual process leads only to frustration.

Once the plan has been revised and facility employees have been retrained, another drill should be held. This should have as one of its primary objectives the testing of revisions to the plan and/or manual for their appropriateness and efficiency. Subsequent critique sessions should reveal any further problems with the revised segments.

LEARNING FROM THE TRAINING EXPERIENCE

The purpose of preparedness training is to ready personnel for specific activities during a disaster and to clarify and increase the effectiveness of procedures for disaster response. Evaluation of such training has a threefold purpose:

1. to provide trainees with feedback about their performance
2. to use that feedback as reinforcement for learning
3. to assess the effectiveness of the training event.

One reliable method of program/training evaluation is to use pretests, posttests, and structured observations. Various training competencies and evaluation techniques are identified in Table 5–5.

Whether the technique used involves, for example, rating scales given to drill auditors or objective examinations completed by trainees, evaluation of program success and behavioral change is difficult. A basic problem in evaluation is use of methods and criteria that measure actual learning.

Although attendance at training programs is *requisite* to learning, it does not *assure* learning. While participation is more likely to result in retention of new information and adoption of new skills, however, learning is enhanced if trainees have the opportunity to actually perform required skills (see Figure 5–4). Multiple-choice objective examinations in conjunction with demonstrations documented by a skills profile of expected competencies are ideal evaluation tools. Multiple-choice exams are less ambiguous than fill-in and true/false exams and are particularly helpful if items are referenced from lecture material. (See Appendix 5–C for principles for preparing multiple-choice items.)

Table 5-5 Example of Training Competencies and Evaluation Techniques

Learning Expected As a Result of Training	Competence Expected as a Result of Training	Possible Evaluation Techniques	Evaluation Method
Application of Knowledge/Skills	Ability to: • Acquire concepts • Recall facts • Recall facts with comprehension • Solve problem(s) • Apply concepts to work settings • Follow directives and procedures • Demonstrate use of equipment or process	Objective tests Rating scales Checklists Behavior in simulations or drills Informal debriefing(s) Subjective tests and feedback Contribution records	Self-pretests and posttests, group, drill auditor, technical consultants, provider/consumer observers
Behavior on the Job	Willingness to: • Attend training events • Complete assignments • Change attitudes/values vis-à-vis disaster preparedness • Practice methods learned in training events • Change procedures • Explain preparedness needs and procedures to peers and subordinates • Use equipment and disaster manual	Rating scales, attendance rosters Interviews Questionnaires Simulations or drills Completion of forms, reports, etc. Handling of patients, personnel, etc.	Drill auditors, supervisors, self, peers

Figure 5–4 Learning Model

Attendance at a program		Participation (e.g., opportunity for dialogue)		Integration on the job (e.g., opportunity for recall and repractice)

REWARDS FOR BEHAVIOR

While attendance alone should not be the only criterion of training adequacy, it does indicate intent to learn. Some facilities specify minimum attendance (i.e., must attend at least 75 percent of all formal programs). However, failure to attend disaster preparedness classes and drills, as in the case of any required employee behavior, should be placed as an anecdotal note in the personnel file and discussed in performance appraisal sessions. Otherwise, preparedness will not be identified as a serious issue. The best indicator of preparedness is consistent and adequate performance in drills and/or real events.

Tests, observer rating schedules, etc., should be valid, i.e., should measure what they are intended to measure, and reliable, i.e., responded to in the same way by different people. These instruments should specify responses stipulated in the plan or manual. For example, if the Central Service supervisor is required to send the triage supply cart to the Triage Area, a valid measure of performance is that the task is documented on a progressive audit form. An indicator of a reliable measure is that many observers working independently are able to use the same audit form to document the same behavior.

One practical way to develop performance criteria is to ask supervisors, staff members, and disaster trainers to define minimum competencies they would expect of participants in a disaster response.

The evaluation process must be viewed as supportive rather than punitive and as an extension of the training experience. Anything that will minimize embarrassment and maximize learning will benefit adult participants. Most adults will become alienated if their performance is criticized openly by evaluators or peers. If they feel castigated (whether justified or not) they may drop out, seeing the experience as potentially punishing rather than rewarding.

Coaching is a widely used method for reinforcing learning in industry, although it has been used less widely in health care settings. This method consists of two components: trainee counseling and guided practice. Coaching is more likely to succeed in changing behavior if it:

1. provides individualized attention
2. proceeds after the employee has been told what behavior is expected

3. encourages employees to use their own "style" of doing things, within defined parameters
4. is not accompanied by threats or punishment
5. involves coaches who are positive and express confidence in the employees' ability (people expected to perform tend to do so)
6. promotes the desire of employees to perform as expected because it accentuates the importance of their roles.

Adults respond better to evaluators who treat them as competent individuals while providing guidance in performance of a skill. Allowing them reasonable flexibility and choice wherever possible enhances their willingness to participate in training and learning. If deficiencies in performance occur, feedback should be tied to expected and actual behavior and not to the learner as an individual. Finally, selective rewards, contingent on specific performance, are superior to rewards for routine performance. If rewards become the norm, they tend to lose their reinforcement power.

The following four case examples illustrate problems in preparedness training and personnel evaluation.

Case #1

Bill W. is a respiratory therapist assigned to work with one other therapist on the evening shift. During a disaster one therapist is expected to respond immediately to the ED and to remain there. The other therapist continues providing care in the facility and initiates a callback of therapists if needed.

A drill was scheduled and widely publicized several weeks in advance. The purpose was to test the full response capability of the ED. The drill scenario called for the simultaneous arrival of multiple burn victims.

Bill arrived in the ED a documented 15 minutes after the drill began. Instead of starting work according to his Disaster Action Card, he began socializing with patients in the ED and doing as little of his prescribed activities as possible. After the drill, Bill complained to several employees that the drill had interrupted his patient rounds schedule and was a "joke."

By not performing actively in the drill but instead engaging in inappropriate activities, Bill did not have to utilize disaster-related skills and knowledge. However, he was present at the informal critique immediately after the drill and contributed suggestions. He also attended the formal critique and provided his department's analysis of the event, which essentially was his opinion and not based on audit criteria. Even so, Bill was commended for his participation in the drill and in the critique sessions.

Discussion

This example identifies two key issues: the need for objective observer audit during drills, and the reward of nonperformance. Had an objective observer been on the scene in the ED, Bill would not have been able to continue his behavior. The ED staff was too busy to keep an eye on him and the fleeting frustration about his noninvolvement was soon forgotten. Staff persons were not aware of his supervisor's commendation for participation and were not asked for input before the reward was given.

Because Bill's nonperformance was rewarded, it is unlikely that he will behave differently in the future, all things remaining constant. He has learned to manipulate the system, do nothing, and learn nothing, yet still receive positive rewards. Bill does not require more learning opportunities—in fact, his skills may be satisfactory, should he choose to practice them. What Bill will require in the future is evaluation of performance by objective criteria, with accurate feedback.

Case #2

After a surprise inspection by the fire marshal, the SNF administrator announced to a meeting of area managers that fire drills were to be held monthly "until people learn what they are supposed to do." After that, the SNF had four surprise fire drills in as many months. However, the drills frightened patients and, after the second one, the staff became demoralized. The drills came to an abrupt end when a patient's family filed a complaint with the State Nursing Home Commission.

Discussion

In this case, drills were the primary learning tool. But deficiencies identified during them never were defined and personnel remained largely untrained and their behavior unchanged. The constant use of the same scenario, the frequency of the drills, and their negative impact on patient care all were considered punitive and unreasonable by personnel, although their sentiments were ignored. The drills would have continued if a patient had not complained.

An inflexible approach to disaster preparedness training will not foster learning. Instead, it will generate resistance. If participants do not know what is expected of them and how to perform, no amount of drilling will change their behavior, either in a drill or in a real disaster.

Case #3

In this real disaster, an ED received only ten minutes' warning before ten victims arrived in three rescue vehicles. Triage was not opened, no written assessment of staffing needs was made, and no callbacks were begun. The house supervisor was notified just as the victims began arriving.

Three critical patients were in the ED at the time of the initial notification. Five other patients were waiting to be seen, one was waiting for admission, and three were in the process of examination. One nurse had been "floated in" from orthopedics to fill in for an ED nurse who had called in sick, and personnel at the moment were barely able to handle existing patients effectively. The supervisor was "paged" as soon as notification of the disaster was received but failed to respond because the page system could not be heard in Medical Records, where she had gone to retrieve a patient file. In a postdisaster critique, Nursing Administration arranged for the ED charge nurse on duty at the time to attend the entire disaster preparedness orientation program again, and she received a verbal warning about poor judgment.

Discussion

The major impediment to response was not the ED charge nurse's lack of training, but a number of other factors. The ED *Disaster Manual* was locked in the ED director's office because it was undergoing revision. The callback work sheet was not located where it should have been (it had not been replaced after a previous drill). Also, notification delay also contributed to the charge nurse's inability to mobilize staff in time. All these elements clearly were out of the nurse's control. Requiring that he or she be retrained, given the actual circumstances, seems inappropriate.

What this case demonstrates is that on occasion individuals perform poorly not because they are untrained but because there simply are too many obstacles that preclude appropriate action. This situation may repeat itself unless criteria for judging the extent to which performance deviates from expectations are developed. It also may prove necessary to revise the plan in order to prevent similar occurrences in other situations. Tabletop and paper drills are useful methods for highlighting problems such as these. The drills can be used to introduce contingency factors and enable personnel to improvise and be more flexible when they encounter new problems. Probably the most vital point illustrated by this case is the need for a revision of the written plan. The events that took place were largely procedural, rather than deficiencies in personnel skills or judgment.

Case #4

Carol J. responded to a drill callback wearing street clothes. She had been called because she was a member of the next oncoming shift. Because she responded in street clothes, she had to return home afterward to change into her uniform. This resulted in her being 30 minutes late for the scheduled shift change and also meant that a day-shift nurse had to fill Carol's slot until she returned. This tardiness was one of several during the past month. Carol received negative feedback from the off-going staff member, who was tired and frustrated at having to stay late. Carol's supervisor also counseled her about her tardiness record. In addition, at the next staff meeting a comment was made about excessive overtime in the unit.

Discussion

Carol's tardiness before the drill and as a result of the drill are separate issues. It is essential that personnel not be punished for making attempts to meet expectations. In this circumstance it is doubtful anyone so criticized would be willing to participate in future drills. The way in which Carol was treated probably will generate anger and resentment; it will not improve or assure future performance.

SUMMARY

Training is fundamental to disaster preparedness. It gives planners the opportunity to evaluate the disaster plan and the manual carefully and gives personnel a low-risk context for learning and practice.

Practice and the freedom to critique a learning experience are essential to adult education. Teaching is likened to traditional settings, where the student is assumed to be passive but nonetheless amenable to the teacher's prowess. Adult education makes the opposite assumption—that adults learn best when they are able to practice, to compare new information and/or skills with their prior experience, and when they are active participants in the educational event. The focus of adult education therefore is on methods as much as it is on content.

Disaster preparedness training should be based on adult education concepts. Preparedness training:

1. provides skills practice as a complement to cognitive learning
2. involves the learner in translating procedures on paper into action
3. builds self-esteem and confidence in learning by providing timely feedback on performance

4. promotes interdependence in collegial relationships and independence of judgment.

A 12-month training plan, presented as a framework for developing training programs, has four components: a core program, quarterly core programs, training-of-trainers, and practice situations at unit and/or department levels designed to prepare personnel to implement the disaster plan. These practice situations also provide a means for evaluating plan and/or manual efficacy.

While participation in a large-scale mock-casualty exercise has many advantages, the disadvantages suggest withholding such an event until after core training and smaller programs and drills have been conducted. The considerable effort expended in a large-scale drill will then be rewarded when personnel, prepared by methodical training, function appropriately.

The plan and manual, tested by drills, is likely to require revisions after any exercise. Therefore, systematic critiquing is a vital evaluation tool. Once problems are identified, a timetable for revisions should be established to ensure timely change. The cycle should be repeated as retraining for the revisions takes place.

NOTES

1. Joint Commission on Accreditation of Hospitals, *Accreditation Manual for Hospital, 1985* (Chicago: Author, 1985), 132–133.

2. *Assessing Your External Disaster Plan and Disaster Drills*. Hospital Council of Southern California, Office of Professional Services, 1983, 65.

3. Ibid., 72.

4. Ibid., 75.

5. Alexander M. Butmon, *Responding to the Mass Casualty Incident: A Guide for EMS Personnel.* (Hartford: Educational Direction, Inc., 1982), Chapter 13.

6. Gary Morris, "Myths of Mass Casualty Training," *Journal of Emergency Medical Services* 9, no. 4 (April 1984).

REFERENCES

Bergevin, P.; Morris, D.; and Smith, R. *Adult Education Procedures.* New York: Seabury Press, 1966.

Bramer, L. *The Helping Relationship.* Englewood Cliffs, NJ: Prentice-Hall, 1973, 47–170.

Broadwell, Martin. *The Supervisor As Instructor.* Reading, MA: Addison-Wesley, 1970.

Brown, F. Gerald. *Assessing Training Needs.* Washington, DC: National Training and Development Services Press, 1974, 5–46.

Burke, Warner, and Beckhard, Richard. *Conference Planning.* Washington, DC: National Training Laboratory Institute for Applied Behavioral Science, National Education Association, 1970.

Cormier, L. Sherilyn; Cormier, William; and Weisser, Roland. *Interviewing and Helping Skills for Health Professionals.* Monterey, CA: Wadsworth Publishing Co., 1984, 15–45.

Gardner, Neely. *Group Leadership*. Washington, DC: National Training and Development Service Press, 1974, 91–116.

Haggard, A. "A Disaster Game That Prepares You for the Real Thing." *RN* 47, no. 10 (October 1984): 22.

Herman, R. "Disaster Preparation—Developing a Plan." *Emergency* 15, no. 1 (January 1983): 28.

Kanfer, Frederick, and Goldstein, Arnold (eds.). *Helping People Change*. New York: Pergamon Press, 1975, 117–194.

Klinzing, Dennis, and Klinzing, Dene. *Communication for Allied Health Professionals*. Dubuque, IA: Wm. C. Brown, 1985, 103–194.

McConnell, Charles. *Managing the Health Care Professional*. Rockville, MD: Aspen Systems Corporation, 1984.

McMullen, J., and May, R. "Operation Campbell: A Disaster Exercise." *Emergency* 17, no. 2 (February 1985): 30.

Sampson, Edward and Marthas, Marya. *Group Process for the Health Professions*. New York: John Wiley and Sons, 1981, 3–26.

Appendix 5–A

Characteristics of Selected Training Methods

Method	Description	Advantages	Disadvantages
Lecture	A talk by a single speaker to a group. May or may not be followed by question-and-answer session. Usually somewhat formal.	Familiar, flexible, easy to arrange Organized and systematic way of presenting material Can reach a large number of people in short time Assures uniformity of information giving Especially useful for • giving new facts or information lacked by group • stimulating interest • supplementing or stressing materials read • summarizing results of group activities	Difficult to find dynamic speakers with adequate subject-matter knowledge Speaker can't always judge accurately group members' understanding and reaction Can be tiring to group, especially if long Limited opportunity for group participation Not very suitable for controversial subjects or for teaching human relations skills

Source: Reprinted from *A Catalog of Training Materials*, pp. 6–10, U.S. Office of Personnel Management, Washington, D.C., 1957.

215

Method	Description	Advantages	Disadvantages
Conference	Discussion by group members, usually under leadership of a chairperson (often one chosen by the group) who • introduces subject • gets discussion started • helps keep it on the track • sums up, and • closes discussion	Pools ideas, information, and knowledge from many sources If well conducted, permits anybody in group who can do so to contribute Stimulates thinking, ability to work together in groups Especially useful for • exploring problems to which answers are not known • developing new philosophy or approach • developing different aspects of a problem	Practical only if group members have some knowledge of or experience with subject Practical only with small groups Not efficient for organized presentation of new subject matter Requires more time to cover subject Can get ''off the beam'' Good conference leading can be difficult with certain groups and certain personalities
Seminar	Group discussion or exploration, by highly experienced people working under minimum formal leadership, of subject to which ready answers are not available.	Same as for conference Especially useful for situations in which there is no predetermined solution	Requires even more subject-matter knowledge on part of members than does the conference Practical only with small groups Not appropriate for presenting known subject-matter

		Can get "off the beam" Some participants may dominate
Forum	Brief presentation by a speaker, followed by group response with questions, opinions, evaluations, or recommendations Does not attempt to arrive at common conclusion	Free, open discussion by group Development of many different points of view Stimulating, thought provoking Can reach large number of people in short time Especially useful for exploring and for broadening information	Everybody who wishes to talk may not have a chance to do so May be so inconclusive as to be dissatisfying to some people May develop arguments between group members holding conflicting views Contributions may be somewhat superficial and disorganized
Symposium or Panel	Presentation (often including conflicting views) by small group of speakers, followed by questions from audience	Can reach large number of people in short time Fast pace and change in speakers hold interest Brings knowledge from number of sources to bear on subject Spotlights issues Brings out opposite views Stimulates thinking and analysis	Requires very careful advance preparation to ensure adequate coverage, coordination, integration Limited in general to views of the speakers Can easily get "off the beam" Provides only limited participation by group members

Method	Description	Advantages	Disadvantages
Case Study	Group discussion of a preselected case history, under direction of a discussion leader. The case may be presented orally, in writing, in pictures, or on records	Permits participation by all members of group Interesting to group members Brings knowledge from number of sources to bear on the subject Develops independent thinking and analytical skill Develops problem-solving ability Develops insight and understanding Gives members a chance to test their ideas with others Affords opportunity to work with others	Requires small groups Requires skillful leadership, familiar with case and well-grounded in subject involved in case Takes considerable amount of time In some instances, requires extensive advance study of cases by group members Suitable case materials are not always available
Incident Process	Same as above, except discussion starts with an incident—such as a worker's refusal to work overtime—and group has to develop, by questioning the leader, facts they would be given in a case study. Group also has to	Same as for case study, plus • Requires no advance study by group members • Develops skills in obtaining facts by questioning • Pressure to "decide on	Requires small groups Requires skillful leadership Takes time Many office situations do not produce dramatic "incidents" that can be used profitably this way Forced decision making may

	define the real issue, something usually done for them in a case study. Often requires group to decide what action they would take to deal with the incident.	action" can develop ability to reconcile differences	create resentment in some members not yet ready to decide
Role-Playing, Skits, Simulated Situations	Case studies and incidents brought to life; members of the group "act out" the case or incident, and group observes and analyzes it	Facilitates understanding and communication despite semantic difficulties Develops social insights and skills Changes attitudes and behavior Permits people to obtain "protected experience" with no penalty for mistakes Provides realistic demonstration of real-life situations Especially useful for human relations training	Requires very skillful leadership Requires careful advance planning (except in spontaneous role-playing) May appear artificial to those unfamiliar with situation portrayed May be painful way of learning for self-conscious participants Difficult to communicate results
Demonstration	Person actually goes through a procedure—actually does it as individual would on the job, so group can see the action carried out correctly	Interesting to group Aids motivation Helps emphasize and clarify important or difficult points Illustrates application of theory or principle Realistic, true to life Emphasizes correct procedure	Requires exceedingly careful preparation and rehearsal to ensure complete, correct coverage All members of a large group may not be able to see well Trainees may miss point unless the purpose of the

Method	Description	Advantages	Disadvantages
			demonstration and things to look for are made clear Some things don't lend themselves to demonstration
Tours, Onsite Inspections	Trainees go to actual site of operation being studied, see first-hand what goes on, where, and under what conditions	Gives vivid, real, first-hand experience Broadens perspective, understanding Increases interest, creates enthusiasm	Requires considerable time, energy, effort to arrange Requires careful planning on part of those to be visited Can be quite tiring, physically, to group members Can be somewhat disruptive to normal work operations Difficult to keep within practical limits
Written Words	Includes textbooks, articles, outline, summaries, notes, instruction sheets, job break-downs, workbooks, manuals, procedures, etc.	Can reach large numbers of people with same information Can be studied at times and under conditions suitable to trainee Usually represent superior expression of ideas and information Words are ultimate means of expressing ideas; printing	Cannot be used to train those who cannot read Same word has different meaning or connotation to different people Difficult to get some people to read except for entertainment Some people don't seem to learn well by reading It's hard and time-consuming

		Advantages	Limitations
		words preserves and facilitates exchange of these ideas Reading is an efficient way of learning; knowledge so acquired probably represents most of the total knowledge of the average person here	work to find and select good materials for trainees to read Training materials often have to be developed specially to be suitable for the purpose intended
Pictures	Includes motion pictures, photographs, cartoons, charts, diagrams, etc.	Add interest Facilitate understanding Focus attention, help trainees remember Reveal hidden, remote, or hard-to-get-at processes or objects Strengthen emotional appeal Provide variety, change of pace Especially useful in training people who cannot read	Trainers tend to rely on them too heavily Entertainment value sometimes interferes with teaching value Can seldom do the whole training job—should be used as aids or supplements Sometimes difficult to integrate properly with other teaching methods and aids Suitable pictures not always available, and some are difficult and expensive to produce Some require expensive, unwieldy equipment, electricity, darkened rooms

Example of Departmental Drill Critique Checklist

- Time Drill Initiated _____ A.M./P.M.
- Time Casualties received _____ A.M./P.M. (Attach Triage Log)
- **Notification**, Administrative Personnel, Emergency Department

  Name _____ Time _____ By Whom _____
  Response _____ Time Arrived _____
  Name _____ Time _____ By Whom _____
  Response _____ Time Arrived _____
  Name _____ Time _____ By Whom _____
  Response _____ Time Arrived _____

- **Notification:** Hospital

  Administration ____ A.M./P.M.   Nursing Office ____ A.M./P.M.
  Surgery ____ A.M./P.M.   X-Ray ____ A.M./P.M.   Lab ____ A.M./P.M.
  ICU ____ A.M./P.M. IV Team ____ A.M./P.M. Blood Bank ____ A.M./P.M.
  Security ____ A.M./P.M.
  Comments:

- **Staff Call-In** (Attach Call-In Roster and Notes)
  Time Initiated ____ A.M./P.M.   By Whom _____
  Comments:

- **Command Post** . . . Emergency Department (Attach Command Post Records)
  Time Opened ____ A.M./P.M.   By Whom _____
  Staff _____
       _____
       _____

Comments:

- **Staff Assignments** (Attach Assignment Sheet from Command Post)
  Comments:

- **Triage**
  Time Established _____ A.M./P.M.
  Medical Officer _____ Time Arrived _____ A.M./P.M.
  Casualty Breakdown (Attach Copy of Tags)
  Comments:

- **Treatment Area** (Major)
  # of Actual ED Patients at Start of Drill _____
  # of Beds Available at Start _____
  # of Staff on Duty at Start _____
  Breakdown: MD __
              RN __
              LVN __
              Tech __
  Comments:

- **Delayed Treatment Area**
  Time Established _____ A.M./P.M.
  Comments:

Summary Sheet:
1. Problems

2. Suggestions

Signature of Evaluator _____
Date _____

Appendix 5–C

Considerations in Preparing
Multiple-Choice Exams

PROFESSIONAL EXAMINATIONS DIVISION

THE PSYCHOLOGICAL CORPORATION · **757 THIRD AVENUE** · **NEW YORK, N. Y. 10017**

SOME PRINCIPLES FOR PREPARING
MULTIPLE-CHOICE ITEMS

The multiple-choice test is the most widely used type of objective examination. It offers so many advantages over other kinds of tests that it is relied upon almost exclusively for testing sizeable groups under standardized conditions.

A multiple-choice test consists of a series of "items." Each item comprises a "stem" and three or more answer choices, or "options." One of the options is correct, while the others ("distracters") are incorrect. The examinee's task is to select the correct option for each item, and his score is based on the number of items he answers correctly.

The preparation of good test items is one of the most exacting and challenging tasks in the field of creative writing. With the possible exception of legal documents, few other words are read with such critical attention to expressed and implied meanings as those in test items. Even experienced item writers have difficulty avoiding serious ambiguities. An editorial review of newly prepared items by at least one other person is almost always necessary.

The following set of principles and illustrations is intended to help item writers avoid some of the pitfalls that frequently lead to defective items. These principles cannot be applied rigidly, because some of them might have to be sacrificed in favor of others. Nevertheless, they do cover many of the problems commonly encountered in item construction. Defects in items can usually be traced to violation of one or more of these principles.

1. **The stem may be in the form of a question or an incomplete statement.**

    These two most common types of multiple-choice items are illustrated below. They differ only in the construction of their stems. Both ways of writing this particular item are acceptable. Some items, however, may be more amenable to one of these formats than to the other.

    Completion Type

    Birmingham, Alabama, is sometimes called the "Pittsburgh of the South" because it is

    1. a steel production center.
    2. an important shipping port.
    3. a textile manufacturing center.
    4. a leading maker of glass.

    Question Type

    Why is Birmingham, Alabama, sometimes called the "Pittsburgh of the South"?

    1. It is a steel production center
    2. It is an important shipping port
    3. It is a textile manufacturing center
    4. It is a leading maker of glass

Note: In the sample items accompanying the statements of principles, the correct option is always number 1. In draft form, options should appear in this order to insure that the correct answer intended is readily identifiable to reviewers. Rearrangement of the options is usually left to the final editing stage.

Source: Reproduced by permission of The Psychological Corporation. All rights reserved.

224

2. The problem or question should be presented clearly in the stem.

The stem should state the problem or question so clearly that a well-informed examinee should be able to anticipate the appropriate answer before he looks at the options. The examinee should not be required to guess the intent of the item writer.

Poor	*Improved*
Washington was	In what year did the State of Washington enter the Union?
1. admitted to statehood in 1889.	1. 1889
2. part of the Territory of Oregon until 1912.	2. 1811
3. made a state in 1811.	3. 1848
4. part of the Northwest Territory until 1848.	4. 1912

Note: The stem in the poor item is ambiguous and could have so many correct predicates that the examinee would have to read the options before he could understand what was being asked. "Washington" could be George Washington, Washington, D. C., the State of Washington, or some other Washington.

3. The correct option should be unequivocally correct and the distracters unequivocally wrong.

Poor	*Improved*
Clouded vision is a symptom of	The most common symptom of cataracts is
1. cataracts.	1. clouded vision.
2. glaucoma.	2. ocular pain.
3. diabetes.	3. double vision.
4. retinal detachment.	4. loss of light perception.

Note: In the poor item, the options are all potentially correct.

4. Both the stem and the options should be as brief and straightforward as possible.

A. Avoid complex sentence structures that make comprehension difficult.

Poor	*Improved*
If two thermometers placed in a room both register 70° F when read an hour later and the bulb of one is then completely covered by a piece of wet cloth, then one would expect that, upon reading the temperature of the two thermometers two hours later, the temperature shown by the thermometer whose bulb was covered would be	If the bulb of one of two thermometers in a warm room is completely covered by a wet cloth, the covered thermometer would show
	1. a lower temperature than the uncovered one.
	2. a higher temperature than the uncovered one.
	3. the same temperature as the uncovered one.
1. lower than that on the uncovered thermometer.	4. either a higher or lower temperature depending on the moisture in the air.
2. higher than that on the uncovered thermometer.	
3. the same as that on the uncovered thermometer.	
4. either higher or lower than that on the uncovered one depending upon the condition of the air in the room.	

B. A positive statement of a problem is preferable to a negative one. Items requiring identification of the option which is NOT in the specified realm or category are undesirable. Examinees may overlook critical terms such as "not" or "except."

Poor	*Improved*
Which of the following countries is not located in Europe?	On which continent is Senegal located?
1. Senegal	1. Africa
2. Greece	2. Asia
3. Poland	3. Europe
4. Finland	4. South America

C. The stem should be restricted to information directly relevant to the question or the statement of the problem.

Poor	*Improved*
The nomination of Cabinet officers is one of many responsibilities of a United States President. Nominations of Cabinet members are ratified by the	Nominations of United States Cabinet members are ratified by the
1. Senate.	1. Senate.
2. House of Representatives.	2. House of Representatives.
3. Joint Chiefs of Staff.	3. Joint Chiefs of Staff.
4. House Judiciary Committee.	4. House Judiciary Committee.

D. The stem should include any words that otherwise would have to be repeated in each option.

Poor	Improved
Water can be changed to steam by	At sea level, water can be changed to steam by heating it to a Fahrenheit temperature of
1. heating it to a temperature of 212°F at sea level.	
2. heating it to a temperature of 100°F at sea level.	1. 212°.
3. heating it to a temperature of 200°F at sea level.	2. 100°.
4. heating it to a temperature of 250°F at sea level.	3. 200°.
	4. 250°.

5. **Options should be parallel in construction and content.** All the options should fit grammatically with the stem, and they should all be plausible answers to only one implied or stated question (how, when, who, where, how many, etc.).

Poor	Improved
Commercial processing of bauxite	The purpose of processing bauxite is to extract
1. produces aluminum.	1. aluminum.
2. requires oil-fired blast furnaces.	2. zinc.
3. occurs mostly in Canada.	3. plastics.
4. is impractical and unprofitable.	4. asbestos.

Note: Nonparallel options most often follow stems which fail to set forth the problem or question clearly in accordance with Principle 2.

6. **Items should not contain cues that might give away the correct answer on extraneous grounds. This type of error includes:**

A. Unusually long, qualified correct options contrasting with short, vague distracters

B. Distracters which fail to complete the stem in good grammatical form

C. Key words appearing in stem and correct option but not in distracters

7. **All the options should be plausible to the intended examinee group.**

A. An option that draws no responses makes no contribution to measurement, and one that draws only a few responses may contribute to errors in measurement.

B. An item should not set forth a condition contrary to known facts thus leaving the examinee in the dilemma of either ignoring erroneous statements or not choosing the desired answer.

8. **Attention should be given to the relative inclusiveness of the stem and the options.**

Poor	Improved
What country is largest?	Which of the following countries has the largest land area?
1. China	
2. Japan	1. China
3. Thailand	2. Japan
4. Korea	3. Thailand
	4. Korea

Note: The poor item neither provides necessary limitations in the stem nor provides the correct answer to a literal reading of the stem. The improved item provides the necessary limitation in the stem, but as in any item of the "Which of the following..." variety, it has the defect that the answer cannot be anticipated without referral to the options.

9. **In an item calling for a judgment, the authority or criterion that is the basis for the correct option should be specified.**

Poor	Improved
The men best suited to rule the state are the	According to Plato, the men best suited to rule the ideal state are the
1. philosophers.	
2. soldiers.	1. philosophers.
3. teachers.	2. soldiers.
4. businessmen.	3. teachers.
	4. businessmen.

Note: This principle is particularly important for items concerned with mastery of "good" practices in a technical or professional field.

10. **"All of these" should never be used as an option. If "all of these" were used as a correct option, all the options for that item could be defended as being correct. As a distracter, it is inconsistent with directions that there is only one correct answer.**

11. **The use of "none of these" as an option is rarely justified.**

   A. If "none of these" is used as a distracter, the correct option should be exactly correct.

Poor	*Improved*
What is the decimal equivalent of ⅟₁₆?	What is the decimal equivalent of ⅟₁₆?
1. .063	1. .0625
2. .125	2. .1250
3. .160	3. .1600
4. None of these	4. None of these

Note: In the poor item, the first option is not exactly correct, therefore "none of these" is defensible as a correct option.

   B. If "none of these" is used in some items, then it should appear as an option in all of the items in that test or section, and it should be the correct answer in a number of items.

   C. "None of these" should not be used if the other options have exhausted the logical possibilities. The item should be discarded or revised instead.

12. **Items of the form "What would you do?" should be avoided, because the correctness of any response could be defended. First- and second-person pronouns should not be used, principally because the referent may be unclear.**

13. **The answers to items should not be subject to change within a short time.**

Poor	*Improved*
Where were the summer Olympics held three years ago?	Where were the summer Olympics held in 1972?
	1. Munich
1. Munich	2. Montreal
2. Montreal	3. Tokyo
3. Tokyo	4. Mexico City
4. Mexico City	

14. **Items should be directed toward important learning objectives. While the evaluation of knowledge of specific facts is often a legitimate measurement goal, testing of trivial knowledge should be avoided.**

Poor	*Improved*
The treaty of Brest-Litovsk was signed by Russia on	The treaty of Brest-Litovsk concerned Russia's territory following
1. March 3, 1918.	
2. March 4, 1918.	1. World War I.
3. April 3, 1918.	2. World War II.
4. April 4, 1918.	3. the Crimean War.
	4. the Russo-Japanese War.

Many texts and pamphlets contain more detailed discussions of the theory and practice of test construction. Several of them should be studied by anyone attempting to design and write tests. Following are four good sources.

Ebel, Robert L. *Essentials of educational measurement.* Englewood Cliffs, N. J.: Prentice-Hall, 1972.

Gronlund, Norman E. *Measurement and evaluation in teaching.* Second edition. New York: Macmillan, 1971.

Gronlund, Norman E. *Constructing achievement tests.* Englewood Cliffs, N. J.: Prentice-Hall, 1968.

Thorndike, Robert L. and Hagen, Elizabeth P. *Measurement and evaluation in psychology and education.* Third edition. New York: Wiley, 1969.

Chapter 6

Epilogue

Disasters are disruptive to facility operations, to community and family structures, and to individuals. They can and do change lives, sometimes permanently. An event of any scale has the potential for touching thousands of people and leaving a lasting impact on community values and the way in which people view society and their place in it.

A disaster event always evokes emotional response. Some people internalize the experience; others externalize it. For some it accentuates self-doubt and guilt while others see a disaster event as catalytic and as an opportunity for change. When it comes to the emotional impact of disaster, no one emerges unscathed. Health care personnel are as much at risk as anyone else.

DISASTER STRESS SYNDROME

Because they are sudden and their scope is impossible to predict, disasters cause unexpected emotional and somatic health changes. Reactions are wholly personal.

"Death imprint" is especially characteristic of disaster reactions. Preoccupation with thoughts of the disaster and of death are common. The survivor relives the disaster through vivid nightmares and intrusive daydreams. Environmental stimuli may trigger flashbacks of the disaster. These thoughts often interfere with normal functioning and productivity. Increased awareness of the fragility of life is common. Some survivors adopt an attitude that since life may be snuffed out at any time, "Let's live life to the fullest." Others adopt an attitude that since life is so fragile, "Let's protect it as much as possible." The latter group may become overly cautious in their life or overprotective of their loved ones.[1]

229

Disasters can have short- and long-term effects. The following is a partial list of psychological and physiological indicators:

Psychological	*Physiological*
aggression	chest pain
aimless walking/running	crying
alcohol and drug use	fatigue
amnesia	gastrointestinal distress
anger	headaches
antisocial behavior	hypertension
anxiety	hyperventilation
bargaining	insomnia
blaming others	loss of appetite
combativeness	muscle weakness
confusion	nightmares
denial	palpitations
depression	preexisting conditions
distractibility	exacerbated, (e.g.,
fear	asthma, diabetes)
hysteria	skin eruptions
irritability	startle reactions
loss of interest in loved ones	sweating
panic	tremors
social isolation	
withdrawal	

These responses are functional coping mechanisms. While some people recover quickly, for others the experience can last for years. Disaster planners should assume that any personnel directly involved in facility response (be they in triage, treatment, or support roles) will experience some level of emotional or somatic stress symptoms.

VICTIM RESPONSE

A disaster can be as devastating for those who witness it but are not physically harmed as it is for the primary victim. Persons "skipped over" by a tornado while their neighbors' homes are destroyed, those who "missed the plane" and the air crash that followed, and the person who "left before it happened" are examples of secondary but nonetheless real victims. In documenting individual reactions to a devastating flood, a community mental health center in California identified seven categories of responses and useful interventions (Table 6–1).

Table 6–1 Seven Categories of Victim Reaction and Useful Interventions

Category	Selected Interventions
1. GRIEF: denial, anger, depression	Farewell rituals for coping with loss of homes, family members, pets
2. GUILT: people wondered why their loss wasn't as great as that of others	Counseling
3. ISOLATION: alienation from nonvictims	Victim support groups
4. ANGER: blaming others (government, insurance companies)	Psychotherapy; assistance in letter writing
5. DEPRESSION	Problem-solving oriented psychotherapy
6. ANXIETY AND VULNERABILITY	Stress reduction techniques
7. RELATIONSHIP PROBLEMS	Couples therapy focusing on communication skills

HANDLING THE NEEDS OF HEALTH PERSONNEL

Mental health consultation and services are important resources that should be integrated into any planned response to disaster. Facilities anticipating this need designate psychiatrists, psychologists, social workers, and other mental health care professionals for postdisaster assistance. Some facilities tap their own personnel for this role while others contract with external mental health specialists to respond on an as-needed basis.

Once the facility begins responding to a disaster, it also should begin implementing a Critical Incident Stress Debriefing (CISD) process for its personnel. CISD is a stress intervention mechanism aimed at helping personnel to handle better the emotional impact of a disaster event. Mitchell[2] identifies several types, starting if necessary, while the response is under way.

On-the-Scene or Near-Scene Debriefing CISD

This CISD is brief and informal. Its purpose is to help personnel verbalize their immediate feelings. It is conducted by a trained facilitator who meets with individuals during break periods while response to the disaster is in progress. The facilitator must be skilled at group process and well versed for the CISD assignment but need not be a mental health professional.

Initial Defusing CISD

Usually in a group setting, this CISD can be led by a mental health professional or unit supervisor with prior training for the role. Defusing is held within hours of the incident to enable rescuers and treatment personnel to share their feelings and reactions.

Formal CISD

This CISD takes place 24 to 48 hours after the end of an incident. It should be led by a mental health professional skilled in group dynamics and should be mandatory for all personnel. The format for a formal CISD involves five phases:

1. Introductory Phase

The facilitator begins with a self-introduction, then describes the rules of the process. The need for absolute confidentiality is carefully explained. Members are encouraged to make a pact with each other to be silent forever regarding details of the debriefing, especially any details that could be associated with any particular individual. Participants in a debriefing need to be assured that the open discussion of their feelings will in no way be used against them under any circumstances.

2. The Fact Phase

Most facilitators begin this phase by asking the participants to describe some facts about themselves, the incident, and their activities during it. They are asked to state who they are, their rank, where they were, what they heard, saw, smelled, and did as they worked in and around the incident. Each person takes a turn adding details to make the whole incident come to life again in the CISD room.

3. The Feeling Phase

Once all participants have shared sufficient factual information to bring the incident into vivid memory, the facilitator begins to ask feeling-oriented questions. "How did you feel when that happened?" "How are you feeling now?" "Have you ever felt anything like that in your life before?" Again, each person in the room gets a chance to answer these and a variety of other questions regarding their feelings. At times, the facilitator has to do very little. People start talking and the process continues with only limited guidance.

What is important under these circumstances is that the facilitator makes certain that no one is left out and that no one dominates the discussion at the expense of others. Most often participants discuss their fears, anxieties, concerns, feelings of guilt, frustration, anger, and ambivalence. All feelings, positive or negative, are important and should be encouraged.

4. The Symptom Phase

This phase of the debriefing primarily involves answering questions such as, "What unusual things did you experience at the time of the incident?" "What unusual things are you experiencing now?'' ''Has your life changed in any way since the incident?'' and so on. The participants are urged to discuss what is going on now in their homes and in their jobs as a result of their activities.

5. The Reentry Phase

This final phase seeks to wrap up loose ends, answer unresolved questions, provide final reassurances, and develop a plan of action. Summary comments are offered and the participants are advised about getting additional help should they need it.[3] Groups often need a direction or specific activity after a debriefing and this is an opportune time to work out a responsive plan. For example, one situation in which a drunk driver killed several persons was dealt with in the following manner: Health and safety personnel agreed to appear in court at the defendant's trial in full uniform as a form of protest against light sentences for drunk driving. This plan gave them a sense of purpose and unity and was a constructive way to work out their anger and frustration.

CISD should not be used to critique the disaster response. Rather, its purpose is to provide participants with a therapeutic peer counseling experience designed to reduce the deleterious impact of the disaster. Debriefing is a recognition of the emotional needs of personnel.

In addition to CISD, one expert offers a ten-point list of important do's and don'ts for helping personnel to cope emotionally.

1. *Do* remember that recovery after a disaster often takes several years.
2. *Do* provide anticipatory guidance. Discuss the phases of reactions to disaster and the various symptoms. Help the survivor to accept that what the survivor is experiencing is a normal response. If possible, arrange to have the survivor talk with another survivor.
3. *Do* encourage the use of the survivor's own natural support systems—family, friends, peers, clergy. Let the survivor know that it is all right to lean on others for a while.
4. *Do* encourage use of community support systems, such as disaster debriefing sessions, disaster support groups, and mental health center programs.
5. *Do* assist the survivor to face the reality of the event and its consequences; e.g., co-workers may need to have you accompany them to the scene of the disaster in order to overcome their fear.
6. *Do* make a referral for professional counseling or hospitalization if the survivor has persistent thoughts of suicide, is psychotic, is

immobilized, uses self-destructive behavior, or if other interventions have been ineffective.

7. *Don't* use cliches or euphemisms such as "It's God's will," "It's all for the best," or "Well, at least you're alive."

8. *Don't* expect all survivors to react similarly.

9. *Don't* expect a simple cure for the survivor's distress.

10. *Don't* encourage stoicism. Encouraging the survivor to remain strong, to keep in control, and not to express feelings inhibits normal resolution of the disaster experience.[4]

EMERGING TRENDS IN DISASTER EXPERIENCES

Health care facilities are affected by and are a part of the complexity of contemporary life. A traffic accident that spills chemicals or radioactive materials miles from a facility can affect it as surely as an incident on its own grounds. Health care institutions are vulnerable. Their technology, the interdependence of their personnel, and the relative helplessness of their patients make them not just a resource but a potential victim.

Most counties have Emergency Medical Services Systems (EMSS) that link facilities with public safety agencies as well as with state and federal disaster preparedness organizations. As much as possible, facility disaster planning should be integrated with local EMSS plans. Benefits include improved communication, agency coordination, opportunity for joint training programs, and opportunities for large-scale drills. The disadvantage of not doing so is that in the event of a disaster, the institution's response capabilities may be significantly reduced or impaired.

Since the early 1980s there has been a pronounced effort, albeit primarily in urban areas, to create a network of trauma centers. The centers must meet minimum standards established by statute and/or regulations. Trauma centers will not detract from the disaster response of other capable facilities nor from SNF response. Facilities can continue to expect victims from multiple casualty situations close to them or from mass casualty incidents.

How these networks will affect and be affected by disaster response is not yet clear. However, trauma centers no doubt will play a prominent role in the coming years. Generally, large, acute care facilities operating either basic or comprehensive 24-hour emergency services, Level I or II trauma centers all have the capability of managing traumatic injuries resulting from a disaster and will be important resources to disaster planners.

Traditionally, disaster planning in institutions has been reactive rather than anticipatory. Planners have assumed that events would be manageable and familiar, i.e., receipt of victims from an accident, or even evacuation of patients because of a fire in the facility. These are imaginable events—well within the scope of possibility, given a stable social and physical environment. But society is changing dramatically. Disaster planners in the mid and late 1980s must expand the imaginable more than ever before. The following are types of "new" demands that planners should consider.

Scheduled Disasters

A "scheduled disaster" is an event that can be anticipated.[5] Parades, rock concerts, political rallies and marches, and even community picnics have the potential for disaster. In crowd situations, injury and illness are commonplace. But crowds are unique. They afford anonymity. People sometimes behave "differently" in crowds from how they otherwise would, hence what may begin as a small incident can escalate easily and generate numbers of casualties very quickly. The implication for facility disaster planners is the need to inventory scheduled community events, anticipate demands, and update plans accordingly.

One large facility in a southwestern state checks with the police and with park rangers to identify the number of parade and park use permits issued. It updates its callback roster monthly. It knows from experience that what starts out as a peaceful Sunday in the park can end in a melee with dozens injured. The park is frequented by different ethnic groups that meet there for their various national holidays and to compete in soccer games. While this is an obvious example, there are smaller demand situations in every community, whether only once a year for the Mardi Gras or as often as several times a week in some metropolitan neighborhoods.

Another type of scheduled disaster that often is overlooked is weather. In areas where tornadoes or hurricanes are "regular" events, planners should anticipate the potential for disaster.[6] For instance, Texas is tornado country; tornadoes are expected. But when the Wichita Falls area was hit by a series of tornadoes, hospital disaster plans were sorely tested:

> In designing the disaster plan [planners were] prepared for the possibility of approximately 40 victims of a disaster. In reality, there were 579 patients who received treatment, 79 of whom were admitted. So large an increase in number tested the flexibility of the plan. At one point, the hospital ran out of disaster tags and we functioned for 30 to 45 minutes without an adequate method for maintaining an accurate census.[7]

When planning for "scheduled" potential disasters, key questions such as the following may be helpful for updating plans and manuals:

• What "scheduled disasters" are possible in the community this year (e.g., parades, carnivals, severe weather)?
• Do these events have a history of generating casualties? Of what magnitude?
• Does the institution have operational agreements with local EMSS authorities? Do these agreements specify what is expected of the facility in conjunction with community disaster response?
• Is the facility a designated trauma center?
• Do the plan and manual anticipate demand by prescribing a phase-in sequence for gradual response?

Hazardous Substance Disasters

American communities are becoming more vulnerable to hazardous material disasters because more such agents are being transported by truck, rail, and plane. The risk of human, air, water, and soil contamination is ever–present. The impact can be immediate for those who come into direct contact with a substance but some contaminants can remain toxic and in the environment for days or even years. The local EMSS is the best resource to contact for information and assistance, although some facilities, particularly those near petrochemical or nuclear installations, have developed collaborative relationships with those entities. The purpose for doing so is to assure early warning and appropriate response.

The U.S. Department of Transportation operates a 24-hour Chemical Transportation Emergency Center. The Center can be reached toll-free (800) 424–9300 in the continental U.S., and (202) 483–7616 outside, for information concerning hazardous materials and victim treatment.[8]

High–Rise Fires

Larger American cities have had multistoried office and commercial buildings for more than 100 years. But in recent years there has been a marked increase in multistoried residential buildings in small rural communities as well as in urban areas. Many of these are housing complexes for senior citizens. Some communities have witnessed a flurry of high-rise hotel and motel construction as well. The physical landscape has changed and is changing. It is imperative to link facility plans with the possibility of casualties from these high-rise sources.

Since the Las Vegas hotel disasters in the early 1980s, interest has focused on this new problem. How to rescue and treat multiple casualties generated from high-rise fires is beginning to receive a great deal of (belated) consideration. Plans for responses by receiving facilities in a high-rise disaster should assume the need for the following:

- a specific high-rise fire disaster plan that is integrated with the overall EMSS plan for the community
- the capability for handling large numbers of smoke or fumes inhalation and burn victims
- a plan to distribute both ambulatory and critical patients to physicians specializing in family practice, internal medicine and surgery, and reserving the services of pulmonary specialists for consultation.[9]

Even though an institution may not be designated as a receiving facility in a high-rise fire, it may be called upon to provide backup assistance such as receiving inpatients evacuated from receiving hospitals. Interfacility collaboration, planning, and preparedness training are as important for adequate response to this "new age" disaster as it is to any "traditional" incidents.

Computer Vulnerability

Most health care facilities already have computerized patient records, accounts payable/receivable, personnel records, and so forth. Some operate their own large multiterminal mainframe or minicomputers, others use equipment housed elsewhere and access them via telephone lines. Still others use self-contained personal computers (PCs). All of these systems are vulnerable to interruptions of the power supply; unless they are equipped with battery-operated backup power units, a loss in power will mean the loss of data. Needless to say, a computer system that is "down" in a disaster will compound the impact of the event.

Facilities can anticipate this need by storing duplicate copies of software and data in fireproof vaults onsite and off. They also should plan for recovery. In situations in which the mainframe or minicomputer is made inoperable by some event, at least five specialist teams probably will be needed:

1. an operations recovery team to start up equipment and utilities
2. a software recovery team to start up the operating system
3. an input recovery team to start up the input process and restore destroyed data
4. a telecommunications recovery team to reestablish the online system
5. a supplies recovery team to replace forms and documents.

Regardless of the complexity of the computer system, it is essential that its loss be anticipated in the disaster plan. "A good plan . . . covers everything from who gets notified of the disaster to who retrieves the tapes and gets the computer to run them on. The plan should specify step-by-step logistics for recovery, including details on what each staff member is responsible for and when."[10]

Terrorism

Terrorist activity has become an everyday news item—a lone deranged gunman shooting at people from a window is no less a terrorist than someone threatening to blow up a bus for a political cause. Terrorism poses new demands on disaster planners. Facilities may have to receive victims and provide psychological services to police and fire personnel as well. It also is conceivable that a facility may itself become the victim of terrorism. Most institutions include a bomb threat procedure in their planning, but health care facilities in general are unprepared, or underprepared, to respond to terrorism. In fact, there continues to be a significant lack of awareness regarding terrorist motivation and behavior and how to plan a facility response in the event such incidents occur.

All facilities routinely should assess their vulnerability and incorporate their findings into contingency training and tests of the disaster plan. This routine assessment should occur no less than once a year. The political and social climate is a dynamic one. While political hostility may promote organized terrorist acts, economic and social stress may produce deranged and bizarre behavior by individuals. The acting out of either type may be devastating. Watching the climate for changing patterns is essential. Several factors should be considered when developing a terrorism response plan:

- potential for a visit to or use of the facility by prominent political figures and contingencies for managing these situations
- proximity of the facility to political targets, including major waterways, government buildings, ports, and airports
- the number and behavior of known antagonist groups in the community
- response capabilities of the local EMSS to hostage situations and terrorist-related disasters
- expectations of EMSS field personnel and police regarding support from and for health facilities
- the capability of the facility to operate in a self-contained fashion should terrorist activity involve it.

Coordinated collaboration in planning and response among field providers, law enforcement, health facilities, and mental health professionals must be pursued actively. There is no way to predict in today's multicultured, stress-prone, but individual-rights oriented nation what type of event will occur or when. They are occurring and no doubt will continue to do so. Health facilities must be prepared.

Health care institutions will face new challenges in the coming years. Unfortunately, there is widespread pessimism about the capability of health facilities to respond to new-age disasters. A nuclear war is virtually beyond imagination, yet facilities must prepare for nuclear events in spite of the plaint that "All of this planning won't really matter—we probably won't even be here!" Most people, including disaster planners, tend to treat discussions of radiation accidents, terrorism, or nuclear events as something that "won't happen to *us*." They may. In an age where technology, mobility, instant media, and stress overload promote the potential for disaster, no reasonable community or facility can see itself immune or isolated. Survivors will seek help and hope when an event occurs, regardless of the magnitude.

Emergency response capabilities are improving throughout the nation. There are many reasons for this, but foremost among them are (1) the successful growth of EMSS, (2) widespread adoption of disaster response equipment and procedures by paramedic providers, and (3) the development of emergency medicine and nursing and psychotraumatology as specialties.

The authors hope that this work contributes to the philosophy and practice of disaster preparedness, which saves lives and limits loss.

NOTES

1. Alice Sterner Demi and Margaret Shandor Miles. "Understanding Psychologic Reactions to Disaster," *Journal of Emergency Nursing* 9, no. 1 (January/February 1983): 14.

2. Jeffrey Mitchell. "When Disaster Strikes . . . the Critical Incident Stress Debriefing Process," *Journal of Emergency Medical Services* 3, no. 7 (September/October 1980): 36–39.

3. Ibid., 38.

4. Demi and Miles, "Understanding," 15.

5. Jon W. Lowry, George Bey, and Al Carlini. "Responding to a Scheduled Disaster," *Emergency Medical Services* 9, no. 5 (September/October 1980): 17–20.

6. Larry Watson, "Hurricane Alicia: The La Porte Experience," *Emergency* 15, no. 12 (December 1983): 42–46.

7. Callie Seigler-Shelton and Linda Nance Marks, "The Wichita Falls Experience," *Supervisor Nurse* 11, no. 4 (April 1980): 32.

8. Barry D. Smith, "Identifying Hazards," *Emergency* 17, no. 2 (February 1985): 47.

9. Ralph D'Amore, "High Rise Fires," *Emergency* 15, no. 1 (January 1983): 48.

10. Ed Hoag, "Safeguarding Your Computer," *Output* (March 1981): 32.

REFERENCES

Cohen, R.E., and Ahearn, F.L., eds. *Handbook for Mental Health Care of Disaster Victims*. Baltimore: The Johns Hopkins University Press, 1980.

Frederick, C. (ed.). *Training Manual for Human Service Workers in Major Disasters*. Rockville, Md.: National Institute on Mental Health, 1978.

Laube, J. "Psychological Reactions of Nurses in Disaster." *Nursing Research* 22, no. 4 (July-August 1973): 343–47.

McEwen, Michael. "Assessing Emergency Medical Preparedness for Hostage-Taking and Terrorism." *Emergency Medical Services* 9, no. 5 (September/October 1980): 76–77.

Minerd, Rick. "Major Responses of 1984." *Journal of Emergency Medical Services* 10, no. 2 (February 1985): 38–42.

Popkin, Roy. "Crystal Ball Holds Dark Vision for Future Disaster." *Hazard Monthly* (February 1985): 8–9.

Powers, K.A. "Communities in Crisis: Disaster and Unemployment." In *Crisis Counseling,* edited by Ellen Janosik. Monterey, CA: Wadsworth Publishing Co., 1984, 223–39.

Index

A

Action Cards, disaster, 90-92
Action implementation, 44
Action plan detailing, 34-44
  Gantt Timeline chart, 36-37
  PERT Chart, 36, 38-40
  Resource matrix, 43-44
  Responsibility Chart, 40, 42-44
  Scope-of-Work Chart, 34-36
Administration, planning committee
  role, 49
*Administrative Code of the State of
  California*, disaster plan
  standards, 62, 125-128
American Red Cross, 117
Ancillary Service departments, 106-108
  procedures, preparation of, 106-108
Assumed Problem Technique, planning,
  8
Attachments section, 116-120
  cost-recovery procedures, 116-117
  disaster training plan, 116
  long-term disaster response, 117-118
  stress management, 118-120

Authorization letter, disaster manual
  section, 63, 66

B

Bomb threat
  checklist for caller evaluation, 154
  procedures for, sample of, 150-153
Brainstorming, needs assessment, 26
Branch method, planning, 7-8

C

Callback procedure
  callback rosters, 79
  callback worksheet, 77, 78-79
  in disaster manual, 77, 79-80
  physicians and, 79-80
Case study method, training, 218
Casualties
  mass casualty incident, 48-49
  multiple casualty incident, 48
  multiple patient incident, 47-48

Casualty Disposition Log, 89
Centralized planning model, 10-11, 13
Chain of Command, notification and,
    69, 72
Chairperson, planning committee role,
    51-52
Civil Defense authorities, 117
Classical planning, 3
Classroom training, 157-158
Clerk, Triage area, 86
Coaching, training, 208-209
Code definitions, disaster manual,
    67, 70-71
Collaborating agencies, disaster
    manual statement, 67
Command Post section, 80-83
    command post, importance of, 80, 83
    key questions/issues in, 80-83
    opening command post, 83
    procedures, development of, 81-83
    staffing/equipment, 83
Committees, See Planning committee.
Communications section, 86-88
    emergency communication links, 87
    function, 87
    procedures, 88
    staffing/equipment, 87-88
    telephone operations, 87
Community interface section, 113-115
    community interface, disaster
        manual statement, 63, 66, 67
    Media Relations Center procedures,
        113-114
    Public Information Center
        procedures, 114-115
Community involvement, disaster
    planning, 57-59
Comprehensive model
    Assumed Problem Technique, 8
    Off-the-Shelf Technique, 8
    planning, 7
Computer vulnerability disaster, 237
Conference method, training, 216
Core Training Program, 173-175
    curriculum outline for, 174-175
    objectives of, 173
    Quarterly type, 175-176

Cost-recovery procedures, attachments
    section, 116-117
Critical care teams, 103-104
    actors in effectiveness of, 104
    "immediate" victims, care of,
        103-104
    members of, 103
Critical Incident Stress Debriefing,
    231-234
    fact phase, 232
    feeling phase, 232
    formal type, 232-234
    initial defusing, 231-232
    introductory phase, 232
    reentry, 233-234
    symptom phase, 232-233
Critical Path, PERT Chart, 40

D

Damage control, Disaster Manual,
    112-113
Death imprint, 229
Decentralized planning model, 11, 13
Decision-tree, 29
    reverse decision-tree technique,
        29, 31
Delayed Care Area section, 105
    function of, 105
    procedures, 105
    staffing/equipment, 105
Delphi technique, 25-26
Demonstration method, training, 219
Departmental critique form, 90
Departmental responsibilities
    section, 106-109
    Administrative Departments, 108
    Ancillary Service departments,
        106-107
    questions/issues in, 106-108
    security, planning for, 108-109
    Surgical Departments, 106
Disaster
    common types of, 47
    definition of, 47
    minidisaster, 68

Disaster Action Cards, 90-92
　lamination of, 92
　sample, 137-138
Disaster Casualty Disposition Logs,
　sample, 132
Disaster Control Form, sample, 136
Disaster Coordinator, 172, 179
　role of, 51-52
Disaster Initial Notification Form, 89
Disaster manual, 61-122
　attachments section, 116-120
　code definitions/action steps, 67,
　　70-71
　Command Post section, 80-83
　Communications section, 86-88
　Community interface section,
　　113-115
　Delayed Care Area section, 105
　Departmental responsibilities
　　section, 106-109
　documentation section, 88-92
　general guidelines, suggestions
　　for, 120-122
　Internal disaster section, 109-113
　personnel notification section, 69-80
　Personnel Post section, 83-86
　plan implementation section, 63-69
　planning process and, 62
　special incidents section, 115-116
　Treatment area section, 101-105
　Triage section, 92-100
　See also individual sections.
Disaster operations, immediate goals
　of, 53
Disaster planning, 1-15
　branch method, 7-8
　centralized planning, 10-11
　combined centralized/decentralized
　　model, 11, 13
　community resources in, 57-59
　comprehensive model of, 7
　decentralized planning, 11
　facility readiness for, 6
　goals/outcomes of, 62
　incrementalist model of, 7-8
　meaning of, 2-4
　patient-generating criteria, 47-49

planning committee, 13-14, 49-59
prescriptive model of, 8-9
root method, 7-8
strategies of, 4-5
types of, 49, 61
Disaster preparedness
　directive, sample of, 147-149
　drills, 180-205
　training, 157-180
Disaster stress syndrome, 229-230
　Critical Incident Stress Debriefing,
　　231-234
　death imprint, 229
　psychological/physiological
　　indicators, 230
　victim reactions/interventions, 231
Disaster tag, 88-89
　sample tag, 129-130
Documentation section, 88-92
　Area Disaster Personnel/Supplies/
　　Equipment Form, 90
　callback lists, 90
　Casualty Disposition Log, 89
　departmental critique form, 90
　Disaster Action Cards, 90-92
　Disaster Initial Notification Form, 89
　disaster tag, 88-89
　Hourly status reports, 89
　implementation status form, 89-90
　Personnel Assignment Form, 90
　Triage Casualty Logs, 89
Downward evacuation mode, 110
Drills, 180-205
　critiquing the event, 201-205,
　　222-223
　data/site selection, 193
　Disaster Planning Committee role,
　　182-184, 193
　JCAH requirements, 180
　makeup, 198-201
　moulage, 198
　Multiagency Disaster Drill Planning
　　Committee, 192, 193, 195
　objectives of, 192
　paper drills, 186-188
　preannouncement/public
　　announcements of, 195-196

questions in development of, 180-186
revision of plan, 205-206
scenarios for, 183-184, 192-193
simulation board games, 186
staging area selection, 194-195
subsystem drills, 190-192
tabletop drills, 188-190
transportation to, 193-194
value of, 180
"victim" preparation, 196-198
See also Training.

E

Earthquakes, procedures for, sample
of, 155-156
Emergency department
disaster manual elements, 73, 77
stress management, 120
Emergency facility, planning
committee role, 50
Engineering staff, planning
committee role, 50-51
Equipment
Command Post, 83
communications system, 87
Delayed Care Area, 105
Triage Area, 95-96
Equipment form, 90
Evacuation
downward evacuation mode, 110
emergency removal, sample of,
142-146
facility evacuation mode, 111-113
fire procedures, 110
lateral evacuation mode, 110
partial evacuation mode, 110
Evaluation, of plan, 44
Exams, multiple-choice, 224-228
External events
California standards, 125-126
disaster plan and, 49, 61
emergency department and, 73, 77
real/potential danger, determination
of, 73

F

Facility evacuation mode, 111-113
Fire emergencies
California standards, 126-127
evacuation procedures, 110
safety procedures, example of, 141
Five-tier system, triage, 99
Follow-Up Training Programs, 178
Forum method, training, 217
Four-tier system, triage, 99

G

Gantt Timeline Chart, 36-37
Goal/objectives statement, disaster
manual section, 67
Goal setting, 20-22
authority approval for goals, 21-22
goal statements, 21
types of goals, 21
Group size, training groups, 167, 170

H

Hazardous substance disasters, 236
Health facilities
changing planning environment, 9-10
planning difficulties, 4
planning, readiness for, 6
High-rise fires, 236-237
Hourly status reports, 89
sample, 133

I

Imaging-the-need technique, 27-29
steps involved, 28-29
"Immediate" victims
care of, 103
critical care team and, 103-104
Implementation status form, 89-90
sample, 134
Incident process, training, 218-219
Incremental model, planning, 7-8

Internal disaster section, 109-113
  damage control, 112-113
  evacuation procedures, 110-112
  fire procedures, 110
Internal events
  California standards, 126-127
  disaster plan and, 49, 61

J

*Joint Committee on Accreditation of
  Hospitals (JCAH)*, planning
  requirements, 49, 51, 123-124

L

Lateral evacuation mode, 110
Lecture method, training, 215
Life threatening, triage category, 139
Lighting system, California
  standards, 127-128
Long-term disaster response,
  attachment section, 117-118

M

Maintenance staff, planning committee
  role, 50-51
Makeup, 198-201, 202, 203, 204
  blood, preparation of, 200-201
  laceration makeup, 204
  second-degree burns, 202
  simple conditions, simulation of,
    200-201
  supplies for, 199
  third-degree burns, 203
Mandatory training programs, 172
Mass casualty incident, 48-49
Mass casualty programs
  California standards, 125-126
Media Relations Center, procedures,
  development of, 113-114
Medical Records departments,
  procedures, preparation of, 108

Medical staff
  callback procedure, 79-80
  planning committee role, 49
  Triage area, 86
Minidisasters, 68
Most Likely Time, PERT Chart, 39
Moulage, 198
  See also Makeup.
Multiagency Disaster Drill Planning
  Committee, 192, 193, 195
Multiple casualty, 48
Multiple patient incident, 47-48

N

Needs assessment, 22-31
  brainstorming technique for, 24-25
  Delphi technique, 25-26
  imaging-the-need technique, 27-29
  importance of, 22-23
  key questions in, 24
  literature sources, 24
  needs statements, writing of, 23-31
  nominal group technique, 26
  reverse decision tree technique,
    29, 31
  survey technique, 26-27
Nominal group technique, 26
Notification procedure
  disaster manual section, 68-69
  disaster notification form, 76
  phasing, 68-69
  See also Personnel notification
    section.
Nurses
  planning committee role, 50
  Triage area, 86

O

Objective setting, 32-33
  statement of objectives, 32
  verbs used in written objectives,
    32-33
Off-the-Shelf Technique, planning, 8

150-Day Disaster Plan Development and
Plan Review Process, 55-57
Optimistic Time, PERT Chart, 39

P

Paper drills, 186-188
Partial evacuation mode, 110
Patient-generating criteria, 47-49
mass casualty incident, 48-49
multiple casualty incident, 48
multiple patient incident, 47-48
Personnel Assignment Form, 90
sample, 135
Personnel notification section, 69-80
callback procedure, 77, 79-80
Chain of Command, 69-72
notification, steps in, 72-73, 77
Personnel pool section, 83-86
responsibilities of Personnel Pool, 85
staffing/equipment, 85-86
Triage personnel, 86
PERT Chart, 36, 38-41
Critical Path determination, 40
Most Likely Time in, 39
Optimistic Time in, 39
Pessimistic Time in, 39
probability distribution of time,
formula for, 39
Pessimistic Time, PERT Chart, 39
Phasing
example plan, 69
meaning of, 68
Pictures, use in training, 221
Plan implementation section, 63-69
collaborating agencies/facilities
statement, 67
goal/objectives statement, 67
Letter of Authorization in, 63, 66
notification procedure, 68-69
philosophy statement, community/
regional facility, 63, 66, 67
Table of Contents in, 63
terms/decision criteria, 67
Planning
classical planning, 3
health facility difficulties, 4

scientific method of, 3-4
See also Disaster planning.
Planning committee, 49-59
activities of, 52-53
administrative role, 49
chairperson, role of, 51-52
drills, planning of, 182-184
emergency department role, 50
engineering/security/maintenance
role, 50-51
medical staff role, 49
nursing department role, 50
startup checklist, 53-55
Planning process, 17-44
action implementation, 44
action plan detailing, 34-44
goal setting, 20-22
needs assessment, 22-31
objective setting, 32-33
150-Day Disaster Plan Development
and Plan Review Process, 55-57
plan evaluation, 44
problem sensing in, 17-20
relationship to disaster manual, 62
See also individual steps.
Power system, California standards, 127-128
Probability distribution of time,
PERT Chart, 39
Problem-sensing, 17-20
case examples, 18
group-sensing meeting, 19-20
problem indicators, identification
problems, 18-20
Public Information Center
location of, 115
procedures, development of, 114-115
purpose of, 114

Q

Quarterly Core Program, 175-176
Questionnaires, survey technique, 27

R

Rapid treatment diagram, triage, 100
Readi-paks, 96

Reimbursement, cost-recovery, 116
Resource Matrix, 43-44
Responsibility Chart, 40, 42-44
Reverse decision-tree technique, 29, 31
Role playing, training, 218
Root method, planning, 7-8

S

Scenarios, for drills, 183-184
Scheduled disasters, 235-236
Scientific method, of planning, 3-4
Scope-of-Work Chart, 34-36
  components of, 34
Security, Triage Area, 93
Security departments, procedures, preparation of, 109
Security staff, planning committee role, 50-51
Seminar method, training, 216
Simulation board games, 186
Special incidents section, 115-116
Staffing
  Command Post, 83
  communications system, 87-88
  critical care teams, 103-104
  Delayed Care Area, 105
  Personnel Pool, 85-86
  Triage Area, 94
Staging area, drills, 194-195
Status forms
  hourly, 89
  implementation, 89-90
Stress management
  activities for, 118-119
  attachments section, 118-120
  of emergency department personnel, 120
  See also Disaster stress syndrome.
Subelement classes, 178-179
Subsystem drills, 190-192
  mock-casualty exercises, 191
  pre-involvement questions/issues, 191-192
  steps in planning, 190-191

Survey technique, 26-27
  questionnaires, 27
  types of surveys, 26
Symposium/panel method, training, 217

T

Table of Contents, disaster manual section, 63
Tabletop drills, 188-190
  benefits of, 189-190
  materials for, 190
  methodology of, 188
Tagging
  disaster tag, 88-89
  triage, 92-93, 94, 97
Telephone operations
  alternative plan for, 87-88
  breakdown of, 87
Terrorism, 238-239
  response plan considerations, 238
Three-tier system, triage, 99
Training, 157-180
  attendance at events, 171-172
  case study method, 218
  conference method, 216
  content development, 167
  Core Training Program, 173-175
  daily operations barrier, 163
  demonstration method, 219
  Department/Work Unit Programs, 178-179
  evaluation of participants, 208-212
  evaluation of program, 206-207
  Follow-Up Training Programs, 178
  formal classroom/worksite training, 157-158
  forum method, 217
  goals/objectives, development of, 165
  group size, 167, 170
  handout materials in, 158
  incident process, 218-219
  influencing variables, 161
  informal worksite training, 159
  lecture method, 215

mandatory programs, 172
needs assessment and, 165
onsite inspection/tours, 220
organizing program for, 170
personal relevance barrier, 161-162
pictures, use of, 221
"preparedness code" barrier, 162-163
Quarterly Core Programs, 175-176
resources for, 165, 167
rewards for behavior, 198-212
role playing/simulated situations, 219
seminar method, 216
sequence of training program,
    164-171
staff meetings for, 178-179
subelement classes, 178
symposium/panel method, 217
training concepts, 159-160
training methods, 172
Training-of-Trainers Programs,
    177-178
12 month plan, 165
written materials, use of, 220-221
See also Drills.
Training plan, 116
Training-of-Trainers Programs,
    177-178
Transporters, Triage Area, 86, 95
Treatment area section, 101-105
critical care team concept, 103-104
function of, 103
major areas/functions of, 101-102
procedures in, 104-105
questions/issues in, 102
staffing/equipment, 103-104
Triage
meaning of, 92
retriage, 88
serial process of, 92, 140
Triage Area
difference from ED, 92
function of, 94
location of, 93
LVN/ECT role, 94
physical requirements, 93
rating system, 99

readi-paks, use of, 96
security of, 93
staffing/equipment, 94-96
supplies for, 95-96
tagging of casualties, 92-93, 94, 97
time factors, 94
triage cart, 95
Triage Area section
Disaster Manual, 92-100
procedures, statement of, 97-99
questions/issues in, 96-99
rapid treatment diagram, 100
rating system, 99
Triage Casualty Logs, 89
sample, 131
Triage categories, 139-140
delayed, 139
emergent, 139
life threatening, 139
urgent, 140
Triage personnel
clerk, 86
medical officer, 86
nurse, 86
transporter, 86
Two-tier system, triage, 99

U

Urgent, triage category, 140

V

Victim response
Critical Incident Stress
    Debriefing, 231-234
disaster stress syndrome, 229-230
Victims, preparation for drills,
    196-198

W

Weather disasters, disaster preparedness
    directive, sample of, 147-149
Worksite training, 157-158

About the Authors

Jerome Seliger, Ph.D. is Associate Professor of health administration and public health, Department of Health Science, California State University, Northridge. He is also Associate Director of the university's Institute for Communication and Professional Studies. Dr. Seliger's interests are in strategic planning, community health planning and emergency preparedness, and the marketing of community health services. He has nearly twenty years of experience in program and training consultation to organizations as diverse as the USAF, Hawaiian Department of Public Health, U.S. Public Health Service, Dart Industries, Westinghouse and the County of Los Angeles where he acted as principal consultant in the organization of its "public model" Health Systems Agency. Dr. Seliger holds degrees from the University of Minnesota, Southern Illinois University, and the University of Southern California and is co-author of *Delivering Human Services* (Prentice-Hall, 1982).

Joan Kelley Simoneau, RN, is currently administrating the Departments of Ambulatory Care, Emergency Services, and Home Health at Robert F. Kennedy Medical Center, Hawthorne, California. For the past 5 years she has operated a private consulting firm focused on practice, administration, and education in emergency services. Ms. Simoneau has lectured internationally and nationally on topics relating to emergency nursing and disaster preparedness, and served as a consultant to the State of California Department of Health Services in the preparation of the state disaster medical plan, and to the Governor's Earthquake Task Force in planning for state service response to earthquakes of large magnitude.